T0229316

Antimicrobial Stewardship

Editors

PRANITA D. TAMMA
ARJUN SRINIVASAN
SARA E. COSGROVE

INFECTIOUS DISEASE CLINICS OF NORTH AMERICA

www.id.theclinics.com

Consulting Editor
HELEN W. BOUCHER

June 2014 • Volume 28 • Number 2

ELSEVIER

1600 John F. Kennedy Boulevard • Suite 1800 • Philadelphia, Pennsylvania, 19103-2899.
http://www.theclinics.com

INFECTIOUS DISEASE CLINICS OF NORTH AMERICA Volume 28, Number 2
June 2014 ISSN 0891-5520, ISBN-13: 978-0-323-29923-7

Editor: Jessica McCool
Developmental Editor: Donald Mumford

Infectious Disease Clinics of North America (ISSN 0891-5520) is published in March, June, September, and December by Elsevier Inc., 360 Park Avenue South, New York, NY 10010-1710. Periodicals postage paid at New York, NY and additional mailing offices. Subscription prices are $295.00 per year for US individuals, $510.00 per year for US institutions, $145.00 per year for US students, $350.00 per year for Canadian individuals, $638.00 per year for Canadian institutions, $420.00 per year for international individuals, $638.00 per year for international institutions, and $200.00 per year for Canadian and international students. To receive student rate, orders must be accompanied by name of affiliated institution, date of term, and the *signature* of program/ residency coordinator on institution letterhead. Orders will be billed at individual rate until proof of status is received. Foreign air speed delivery is included in all *Clinics* subscription prices. All prices are subject to change without notice. **POSTMASTER**: Send address changes to *Infectious Disease Clinics of North America*, Elsevier Health Sciences Division, Subcription Customer Service, 3251 Riverport Lane, Maryland Heights, MO 63043. **Customer Service: 1-800-654-2452 (US). From outside of the US and Canada, call 1-314-447-8871. Fax: 1-314-447-8029. E-mail: JournalsCustomerService-usa@elsevier.com (print support) or JournalsOnlineSupport-usa@elsevier.com (online support).**

Infectious Disease Clinics of North America is also published in Spanish by Editorial Inter-Médica, Junin 917, 1er A 1113, Buenos Aires, Argentina.

Reprints. For copies of 100 or more, of articles in this publication, please contact the Commercial Reprints Department, Elsevier Inc., 360 Park Avenue South, New York, New York 10010-1710. Tel. 212-633-3874, Fax: 212-633-3820, E-mail: reprints@elsevier.com.

Infectious Disease Clinics of North America is covered in *MEDLINE/PubMed (Index Medicus), Current Contents/ Clinical Medicine, Science Citation Alert, SCISEARCH,* and *Research Alert.*

Contributors

CONSULTING EDITOR

HELEN W. BOUCHER, MD, FIDSA, FACP
Director, Infectious Diseases Fellowship Program; Associate Professor of Medicine, Division of Geographic Medicine and Infectious Diseases, Tufts Medical Center, Boston, Massachusetts

EDITORS

PRANITA D. TAMMA, MD, MHS
Assistant Professor of Pediatrics, Johns Hopkins University School of Medicine, Baltimore, Maryland

ARJUN SRINIVASAN, MD (CAPT, USPHS)
Associate Director for Healthcare Associated Infection Prevention Programs, Division of Healthcare Quality Promotion, The Centers for Disease Control and Prevention, Atlanta, Georgia

SARA E. COSGROVE, MD, MS
Associate Professor of Medicine, Johns Hopkins University School of Medicine, Baltimore, Maryland

AUTHORS

LILIAN M. ABBO, MD
Division of Infectious Diseases, Department of Medicine, University of Miami Miller School of Medicine, Miami, Florida

ELLA J. ARIZA-HEREDIA, MD
Division of Infectious Diseases, Department of Internal Medicine, The University of Texas MD Anderson Cancer Center, Houston, Texas

EDINA AVDIC, PharmD, MBA
Department of Pharmacy, The Johns Hopkins Hospital, Baltimore, Maryland

JOSEPH B. CANTEY, MD
Fellow, Divisions of Pediatric Infectious Disease and Neonatal/Perinatal Medicine, Department of Pediatrics, University of Texas Southwestern Medical Center, Dallas, Texas

KAREN C. CARROLL, MD
Departments of Pathology and Medicine, The Johns Hopkins University School of Medicine, Baltimore, Maryland

ENRIQUE CASTRO-SÁNCHEZ, MPH, RGN
The National Centre for Infection Prevention and Management, Imperial College London, London, United Kingdom

ESMITA CHARANI, MPharm, MSc
The National Centre for Infection Prevention and Management, Imperial College London, London, United Kingdom

NEIL O. FISHMAN, MD
Professor of Medicine; Associate Chief Medical Officer, Healthcare Epidemiology, Infection Prevention and Control, Hospital of the University of Pennsylvania, Philadelphia, Pennsylvania

DEBRA A. GOFF, PharmD, FCCP
Clinical Associate Professor, Infectious Diseases, Department of Pharmacy, The Ohio State University Wexner Medical Center, Columbus, Ohio

KEITH W. HAMILTON, MD
Assistant Professor of Clinical Medicine; Director of Antimicrobial Stewardship, Healthcare Epidemiology, Infection Prevention and Control, Hospital of the University of Pennsylvania, Philadelphia, Pennsylvania

ALISON HOLMES, FRCP, MD, MPH
The National Centre for Infection Prevention and Management, Imperial College London, London, United Kingdom

OMAR M. IBRAHIM, PhD
Visiting Research Scholar, Department of Pharmaceutical Outcomes and Policy, College of Pharmacy, University of Florida, Gainesville, Florida

RAVINA KULLAR, PharmD, MPH
Clinical Scientific Director, Department of Medical Affairs, Cubist Pharmaceuticals, Lexington, Massachusetts

KRISTI KUPER, PharmD, BCPS
GSPC Clinical Pharmacy Manager, VHA Performance Services, Houston, Texas

VERA P. LUTHER, MD
Associate Professor of Medicine, Section on Infectious Diseases, Center for Antimicrobial Utilization Stewardship and Epidemiology, Wake Forest School of Medicine, Wake Forest Baptist Medical Center, Winston-Salem, North Carolina

CHRISTOPHER A. OHL, MD
Professor of Medicine, Section on Infectious Diseases, Center for Antimicrobial Utilization Stewardship and Epidemiology, Wake Forest School of Medicine, Wake Forest Baptist Medical Center, Winston-Salem, North Carolina

SAMEER J. PATEL, MD, MPH
Assistant Professor, Division of Pediatric Infectious Diseases, Department of Pediatrics, Ann & Robert H. Lurie Children's Hospital of Chicago, Northwestern University Feinberg School of Medicine, Chicago, Illinois

RON E. POLK, PharmD, FIDSA, FSHEA
Research Professor, Department of Pharmacotherapy and Outcomes Science, School of Pharmacy, Virginia Commonwealth University/Medical College of Virginia Campus, Richmond, Virginia

SUSAN M. RHEE, MD
Clinical Associate, Division of Infectious Diseases, Johns Hopkins Bayview Medical Center, Baltimore, Maryland

NIMALIE D. STONE, MD, MS
Medical Epidemiologist for Long-term Care, Division of Healthcare Quality Promotion, Centers for Disease Control and Prevention, Atlanta, Georgia

KAVITA K. TRIVEDI, MD
Principal, Trivedi Consults; Adjunct Clinical Assistant Professor of Medicine, Stanford University School of Medicine, Stanford, California

Contents

> Emerging evidence suggests that antimicrobial prescribing behaviors are influenced by local culture and a prescribing etiquette that is abided by all health care professionals. Local cultural unspoken rules often play a more pivotal role than the recommendations of guidelines and policies drawn up by experts in influencing antimicrobial prescribing. It is important to recognize the key drivers of prescribing behaviors and the incentives to alter behaviors and to incorporate these into stewardship programs. This review summarizes key concepts in behavior change in antimicrobial prescribing and the gaps that exist in addressing behavior change in this field.

> Antibiotic stewardship education for health care providers provides a foundation of knowledge and an environment that facilitates and supports optimal antibiotic prescribing. There is a need to extend this education to medical students and health care trainees. Education using passive techniques is modestly effective for increasing prescriber knowledge, whereas education using active techniques is more effective for changing prescribing behavior. Such education has been shown to enhance other antibiotic stewardship interventions. In this review, the need and suggested audience for antibiotic stewardship education are highlighted, and effective education techniques are recommended for increasing knowledge of antibiotics and improving their use.

> Measurement of antimicrobial use before and after an intervention and the associated outcomes are key activities of antimicrobial stewardship programs. In the United States, the recommended metric for aggregate antibiotic use is days of therapy/1000 patient-days. Clinical outcomes, including response to therapy and bacterial resistance, are critical measures but are more difficult to document than economic outcomes. Interhospital benchmarking of risk adjusted antimicrobial use is possible, although several obstacles remain before it can have an impact on patient care. Many challenges for stewardship programs remain, but the methods and science to support their efforts are rapidly evolving.

Collaborative efforts between health care providers with expertise in the diagnosis and treatment of patients with various degrees of immunosuppression are pivotal for the success of antimicrobial stewardship programs in immunocompromised patients.

Inappropriate antimicrobial use and antimicrobial resistance persist across the healthcare continuum. Antimicrobial stewardship guidelines assist healthcare institutions in establishing antimicrobial stewardship programs but rely on infectious diseases expertise and leadership, which are not available in all settings. Despite this, many institutions have found ways to use available resources to perform stewardship activities, with improvements in antimicrobial use and reductions in resistance and cost. This article highlights success stories in nonuniversity hospital settings and proposes antimicrobial stewardship strategies that may be more feasible in settings with limited infectious diseases expertise, information technology, or financial resources.

The successful integration of technology in antimicrobial stewardship programs has made it possible for clinicians to function more efficiently. With government endorsement of electronic health records (EHRs), EHRs and clinical decision support systems (CDSSs) are being used as decision support tools to aid clinicians in efforts to improve antibiotic use. Likewise, medical applications (apps) have provided educational tools easily accessible to clinicians through their mobile devices. In this article, the impact that informatics and technology have had on promoting antibiotic stewardship is described, focusing on EHRs and CDSSs, apps, electronic resources, and social media.

At present, less than half of all acute health care facilities have antimicrobial stewardship programs. By targeting areas that are vulnerable to inappropriate antimicrobial use and by using novel strategies to increase the reach of stewardship interventions, providers can make antimicrobial stewardship a universal practice in all health care settings. This review discusses how stewardship can make large impacts in areas where it has traditionally been absent in facilities both with and without formal antimicrobial stewardship programs.

INFECTIOUS DISEASE CLINICS
OF NORTH AMERICA

Preface

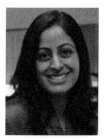 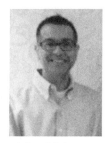 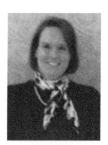

Pranita D. Tamma,
MD, MHS

Arjun Srinivasan,
MD (CAPT, USPHS)

Sara E. Cosgrove,
MD, MS

Editors

The rise in infections caused by antimicrobial-resistant organisms continues to plague us. While resistance genes have been present for millions of years before the advent of modern antibiotics, frequent antibiotic exposure accelerates the emergence of resistance in almost all organisms that cause clinical infections. However, as most of the intuitive targets for antimicrobial agents have been exhausted and as antimicrobial development is not as lucrative as pharmaceutical manufacturers would desire, we are limited in our current antimicrobial treatment options now and in the foreseeable future. Thus, the most realistic, immediate approach is to improve our knowledge and use of existing antimicrobial agents.

Although implementation of antimicrobial stewardship programs across health care facilities is neither incentivized nor nationally mandated in the United States, there are on-going discussions about moving in this direction. Currently, the Centers for Disease Control and Prevention are supporting large studies to move the science of antimicrobial stewardship forward. They are also developing templates to highlight methods to start and expand stewardship programs in health care institutions with a focus on intervention strategies, measurement approaches, and education about resistance and optimal antibiotic use.

In the meantime, as we await policy changes, this issue of *Infectious Disease Clinics of North America* brings together leaders in the field to fill important gaps in knowledge in the world of antimicrobial stewardship, including improving antimicrobial knowledge of prescribers, changing prescriber behavior, utilizing sophisticated research methods and antimicrobial measurement approaches, incorporating novel diagnostic techniques into stewardship activities, and using advanced informatics to enhance stewardship programs. They venture into some nonhospital settings to discuss the role of antimicrobial stewardship, including long-term care facilities, community hospitals, neonatal intensive care units, and oncology and transplant wards. They also discuss innovative methods of improving antimicrobial prescribing practices, such as ward rounds, tackling antibiotic allergies, improving antimicrobial use during transitions of care and at the end of life, transferring some of the work of stewardship onto individual providers, and allocating stewardship resources when resources are limited.

Infect Dis Clin N Am 28 (2014) xi–xii
http://dx.doi.org/10.1016/j.idc.2014.04.001
0891-5520/14/$ – see front matter © 2014 Published by Elsevier Inc.

id.theclinics.com

We thank Dr Helen Boucher for inviting us to develop this issue and the editorial staff of *Infectious Disease Clinics of North America* for all of their assistance. We hope you enjoy reading this issue as much as we enjoyed preparing it.

Pranita D. Tamma, MD, MHS
Johns Hopkins University School of Medicine
600 North Wolfe Street
Baltimore, MD 21287, USA

Arjun Srinivasan, MD (CAPT, USPHS)
Centers for Disease Control and Prevention
1600 Clifton Road
Atlanta, GA 30322, USA

Sara E. Cosgrove, MD, MS
Johns Hopkins University School of Medicine
600 North Wolfe Street
Baltimore, MD 21287, USA

E-mail addresses:
ptamma1@jhmi.edu (P.D. Tamma)
asrinivasan@cdc.gov (A. Srinivasan)
scosgro1@jhmi.edu (S.E. Cosgrove)

The Role of Behavior Change in Antimicrobial Stewardship

Esmita Charani, MPharm, MSc*, Enrique Castro-Sánchez, MPH, RGN,
Alison Holmes, FRCP, MD, MPH

KEYWORDS

- Antimicrobial stewardship • Prescribing behavior • Behavior change • Interventions

KEY POINTS

- Behavioral and cultural determinants influence antimicrobial prescribing.
- Successful implementation of antimicrobial stewardship programs requires recognition of these determinants and the inclusion of the wider health care workforce.
- Hierarchy and leadership within clinical specialties need to be actively involved as part of interventions to influence antimicrobial prescribing.

INTRODUCTION

Antimicrobials are one of the most important therapeutic classes of drugs, with the increasing emergence of resistance threatening their efficacy. Health care institutions are faced with the challenge of treating and preventing infections while reducing the emergence and spread of further resistance. The scientific literature is awash with reports of interventions deployed to address the problem of antimicrobial resistance.[1] Across the globe, concerned public health and governmental institutions are contributing to the debate on how best to tackle antimicrobial resistance by publishing reports, recommendations, and guidance.[2–5]

Despite the emergence of resistance limiting the efficacy of many existing antimicrobial agents and the international interest in this field, there is limited incentive for pharmaceutical companies to invest resources in discovering new antimicrobials.[6] The lack of new agents and increasing resistance to existing therapeutic options means that conservation of antimicrobials is pivotal to current efforts to treat microbial infections alongside interrupting transmission through effective infection prevention.

The authors are supported by the National Institute for Health Research Biomedical Research Centre Funding Scheme at Imperial College (funding number not applicable) and the National Centre for Infection Prevention and Management (CIPM) funded by the United Kingdom Clinical Research Council [UKCRC G0800777].
The National Centre for Infection Prevention and Management, Imperial College London, Hammersmith Campus, Du Cane Road, London W12 ONN, UK
* Corresponding author.
E-mail address: e.charani@imperial.ac.uk

Infect Dis Clin N Am 28 (2014) 169–175
http://dx.doi.org/10.1016/j.idc.2014.01.004
0891-5520/14/$ – see front matter © 2014 Elsevier Inc. All rights reserved.

To this end, antimicrobial stewardship programs aim to give structure and direction to health care institutions trying to adopt a proactive approach to tackling resistance through the prudent use of antimicrobials.

Antimicrobial stewardship describes a host of initiatives designed to optimize the use of diagnostic and laboratory techniques to detect infections and ensure prompt, targeted, and appropriate antimicrobial therapy.[7] Arguably, the aim of all the interventions in antimicrobial stewardship programs is to change behaviors of health care professionals to conserve the efficacy of existing antimicrobial agents while decreasing avoidable harm, including the emergence and transmission of resistance. The focus of this article is on the behavior change elements of antimicrobial stewardship programs.

THE KEY STAKEHOLDERS
The Role of Clinicians

What sets treatment of infections apart from other specialties is the universality of community- and health care–acquired infections. Individuals are at risk of being admitted to a hospital with an infection or acquiring an infection during a health care interaction. The responsibility for the treatment of that infection falls on whichever team of health care providers is responsible for the management of a patient. In many instances, infections are secondary to other medical diagnoses. This means that although medical microbiology and infectious diseases specialties are dedicated to the treatment of infections, in reality health care professionals across all specialties are required to be able to promptly diagnose and treat infections.

Effective stewardship programs should be integrated into existing medical specialties and perhaps led by local noninfection specialist champions. To facilitate acceptance of and adherence to local guidelines implemented as part of a stewardship program, it is necessary to involve opinion leaders within clinical specialties in the development and adoption of evidence-based recommendations. It is important to recognize the factors that will incentivize noninfection specialist health care professionals to change their antimicrobial prescribing behaviors. Research indicates the existence of a set of cultural rules, or a prescribing etiquette, that determines antimicrobial prescribing.[8]

According to these rules, health care professionals adhere to locally drawn lines of authority when it comes to prescribing decisions for their patients and often base decisions on the experience of seniors in their field instead of adhering to antimicrobial stewardship guidelines set by infection specialists.[8,9] This is to be expected because decision making in medicine is reliant on the experience of individual health care professionals, and the interpretation of evidence-based information requires human judgment.[10] Therefore, an incentive to change behaviors in prescribing may be to acknowledge local hierarchies and include opinion leaders within medical specialties in setting up policies and guidelines in prescribing. This is particularly important because not all health care organizations have access to on-site infection specialists and microbiology laboratories. Interventions targeting antimicrobial prescribing behaviors need to be more inclusive and engage with all disciplines within medicine and the wider health care professional workforce.[11]

Engaging Nursing in Antimicrobial Stewardship

Many innovative approaches have been advocated as effective solutions to the problem of delivering health services in areas with limited human resources. The World Health Organization (WHO) task shifting initiative encourages nurses to assume skills and develop roles traditionally held by other professionals.[12] Compelling examples of benefits achieved by these initiatives can be found, particularly in HIV and tuberculosis programs.[13] With adequate training, support, and supervision, nurses can manage complex therapeutic regimens and provide cost-effective, quality care. Thus, it seems logical to take advantage of these experiences and incorporate them within the antimicrobial stewardship agenda.

Currently, the nursing presence in antimicrobial stewardships initiatives remains modest and seems limited to on-the-ground infection prevention and control roles. The implications for the increased involvement of nurses are profound, in particular as their role as organizational knowledge brokers is recognized.[14]

Nurses can serve as repositories of antimicrobial knowledge; they can influence the antimicrobial decisions of other clinicians; and they can collect and evaluate clinical data to inform antimicrobial use.[15] Policy makers and commissioners interested in increasing the involvement of nurses in antimicrobial stewardship programs can adopt different strategies: for example, they can opt to introduce new roles where particularly experienced and highly expert nursing individuals act as antimicrobial stewardship consultants, bridging the evidence regarding optimal antimicrobial use to the nursing sphere of practice, they may also encourage the wider adoption of increased antimicrobial stewardship skills and responsibilities for all nurses, focusing on core competencies acquired, for example, during prequalifying education.

Pharmacists and Antimicrobial Stewardship

The role of hospital pharmacists in antimicrobial stewardship programs needs to be made more prominent on an international level. In some health care settings, the role of the hospital pharmacist in stewardship activities is well established[1,7,8,16]; however, there are still health care systems and models within which pharmacists play a more traditional role and are not integrated into stewardship practices. The knowledge and experience of pharmacists in delivering safety and quality improvement initiatives should be used in the clinical setting to ensure that antimicrobial therapies are prescribed optimally and that stewardship programs are delivered. Pharmacists are pivotal to patient safety pathways and often are in charge of the design and development of decision architectures in prescribing (eg, redesigning medication charts and setting up electronic prescribing systems). Using pharmacy resources across specialties can help augment the organizational efforts in optimizing antimicrobial usage.

To put these staff resources to optimal use, it is important to understand, work with, and shape the cultural and social rules that dictate the dynamics of how health care professionals interact with one another. Across the globe, health care organizations are working in greater multidisciplinary environments, and the key to successful teamwork requires an understanding of the champions and opinion leaders within clinical groups, who can then become engaged in stewardship activities and be encouraged to lead local interventions.[8,9,17]

Patient and Public Involvement

Antimicrobial prescriptions, in community settings, where the bulk of prescribing occurs, are frequently issued in response to demands from patients[18] rather than as clinical necessities. Prescribers may feel the urge to use antimicrobials as a quick and nonconfrontational resource to end a consultation, particularly at times of increased workload and demand, rather than investing time engaging in preventive or educational activities with their patients.

It is essential to equip patients with the necessary skills and confidence to identify when antimicrobials may be inappropriate and alternative self-care measures preferred. Different strategies have attempted to shape patient behavior in relation to antimicrobials. For example, national awareness campaigns have shown a reduction in the volume of antimicrobials demanded by patients.[19,20] If patients are to be empowered to make effective decisions about antimicrobials, interventions need to be mindful of patient perceptions and expectations. For patients' participation to be successful, their need for involvement has to be made clear and adequate support provided to both patients and health care professionals. Support can include educational material, such as leaflets, nonprescription pads, or placebo alternatives to antimicrobials, such as Thailand's Antibiotics Smart Use Program, where, as part of a national stewardship initiative, rather than antimicrobials patients are given an evidence-based herbal remedy for simple colds and coughs.[21]

BEHAVIOR CHANGE INTERVENTIONS

A Cochrane review evaluating interventions to improve antimicrobial prescribing, which included 89 studies from 19 countries, found that a range of interventions has demonstrated success in bringing about improvement in antimicrobial prescribing in hospitals.[1] Overall, restrictive interventions were found more successful in the short term. This review found little evidence, however, comparing different types of interventions, and the majority of studies provided minimal insight into the sustainability and unintended consequences of the interventions described. Furthermore, the studies published to date have not assessed the utility of applying behavior change science to the design, implementation, and evaluation of any interventions antimicrobial prescribing.[1,22] This is while evidence from qualitative studies in antimicrobial prescribing describe the impact of behavioral determinants and etiquette on prescribing.[8,22] Further studies are necessary to evaluate the differences in efficacy between various stewardship interventions and the impact of inclusion of behavior change theory into the development and implementation of interventions. Future systematic reviews in antimicrobial prescribing need to assess interventions against these crucial criteria. To manage the myriad interventions used within stewardship programs, interventions should become a core component of patient safety programs across health care systems.[23] To embed interventions into patient safety programs successfully, there needs to be a greater understanding of the prevailing systems and cultures in order that new interventions are integrated into existing decision architecture and pathways.[24]

The use of technology to change behavior in health care is receiving increased attention.[1] Anything from electronic prescribing to bespoke clinical decision support tools to mobile health systems is currently used in efforts to deliver antimicrobial stewardship interventions. There is no conclusive evidence as to the impact of using different technologies in delivering antimicrobial stewardship programs or the superior efficacy of using these systems over more simple interventions. Although using existing technology has benefits of reaching a bigger audience and easier dissemination of information, technological complexity may hinder uptake of interventions. In the global and local contexts, interventions must be developed to provide information at the lowest level of available technology.

A GLOBAL APPROACH TO STEWARDSHIP

It is important to put the efforts that are carried out in health care organizations into the wider context of the challenge of antimicrobial resistance and health care acquired infections.[2–4] The determinants of antimicrobial prescribing are present at many levels from the local to the global. A majority of the world population does not have access to adequate health care. Stewardship interventions need to take into account human factors and the local cultural and societal determinants of antimicrobial prescribing. Access to and the use of antimicrobials is not standardized across the globe, which is one of the key reasons for the rapid and devastating spread of antimicrobial resistance. To truly tackle the problem, there needs to be a global effort to shift attitudes toward optimizing the use of antimicrobials to conserve their efficacy.

An example of a successful initiative in a resource-limited setting is the accredited drug dispensing outlet model in Tanzania and Uganda whereby nonprofessional practitioners are trained to provide medications and education about these agents in remote areas where few pharmacies exist.[25] This kind of approach across health systems to address antimicrobial stewardship illustrates the systems-thinking approach advocated by the WHO[26] to antimicrobial resistance that takes into consideration the needs of the communities and tries to address the barriers to implementing optimized practice. The key message for all health systems implementing systems to ensure access to effective antimicrobial interventions has to be to look for simple solutions that address local cultures and can be scaled up to become self-sustainable. To address local cultures, there needs to be engagement with the wider frontline health care professional workforce.

In addition, governments should be looking increasingly to introduce strategies to tackle antimicrobial usage not only for human consumption but also for animal consumption. The incentives of antimicrobial usage are different in the agriculture and farming industry, where there is a financial incentive for use of antimicrobials to maximize profits. In these sectors, there needs to be a better understanding of the measures required to incentivize the farming and veterinary industries to change their antimicrobial consumption patterns, which can be done through advocacy, policy change, fiscal measures, and the establishment of minimum standards of practice.

SUMMARY

Emerging evidence suggests that antimicrobial prescribing behaviors are influenced by local culture and a prescribing etiquette that is understood and abided by all health care professionals. The specialist antimicrobial stewardship team model is only one of many approaches. Local cultural unspoken rules often play a more pivotal role than the recommendations of guidelines and policies drawn up by experts in deciding antimicrobial prescribing behaviors. Therefore, to implement successful interventions it is important to recognize the key drivers of prescribing behaviors and the incentives to alter behaviors and to incorporate these into stewardship programs. Additionally, the influence of frontline health care professionals, such as pharmacists and nurses, on antimicrobial prescribing needs to be developed further to increase the effectiveness of stewardship interventions. Antimicrobial stewardship needs to become a core element of patient safety programs in different health care settings. This review summarizes some key concepts in behavior change in antimicrobial prescribing and the gaps that exist in trying to address behavior change in this field. Although the focus is the use of antimicrobials in health care, it is important to not lose sight that antimicrobial use in humans is only part of the larger-scale ecology of antimicrobial resistance. To address stewardship on a global scale, research into the incentives and behavioral determinants of antimicrobial consumption in the veterinary and farming industry needs to be conducted parallel to the work in human medicine.

This research will close the stewardship loop across the different health care settings and sectors.

REFERENCES

1. Davey P, Brown E, Charani E, et al. Interventions to improve antibiotic prescribing practices for hospital inpatients. Cochrane Database Syst Rev 2013;(4):CD003543. http://dx.doi.org/10.1002/14651858.CD003543.pub3.
2. World Health Organisation. The growing threat of antimicrobial resistance. A call for action. 2012. Available at: http://whqlibdoc.who.int/publications/2012/9789241503181_eng.pdf. Accessed February 24, 2014.
3. Centers for Disease Control and Prevention. Antibiotic resistance threats in the United States 2013. Available at: http://www.cdc.gov/drugresistance/threat-report-2013/pdf/ar-threats-2013-508.pdf. Accessed February 24, 2014.
4. G8 Ministers pledge to act on antibiotic resistance. Financial Times 2013. Available at: http://www.ft.com/cms/s/0/172341bc-d428-11e2-a464-00144feab7de.html#axzz2WqdADmif. Accessed February 24, 2014.
5. Ghafur A, Mathai D, Muruganathan A, et al. The Chennai declaration: a road-map to tackle the challenge of antimicrobial resistance. Indian J Cancer 2013; 50:71–3.
6. Boucher H, Talbot GH, Bradley JS, et al. Bad bugs, no drugs! no ESKAPE! an update from the Infectious Diseases Society of America. Clin Infect Dis 2009; 48(1):1–12.
7. Society for Healthcare Epidemiology of America, Infectious Diseases Society of America, Pediatric Infectious Diseases Society. Policy statement on antimicrobial stewardship by the Society for Healthcare Epidemiology of America, Infectious Diseases Society of America, and Pediatric Infectious Diseases Society. Infect Control Hosp Epidemiol 2012;33(4):322–7.
8. Charani E, Castro-Sanchez E, Sevdalis N, et al. Understanding the determinants of antimicrobial prescribing within hospitals: the role of "prescribing etiquette". Clin Infect Dis 2013;57(2):188–96. http://dx.doi.org/10.1093/cid/cit212.
9. Armstrong D, Ogden J. The role of etiquette and experimentation in explaining how doctors change behaviour: a qualitative study. Sociol Health Illn 2006;28:951–68.
10. Atkins L, Smith JA, Kelly MP, et al. The process of developing evidence-based guidance in medicine and public health: a qualitative study of views from the inside. Implement Sci 2013;8(1):101.
11. Charani E, Holmes AH. Antimicrobial stewardship programmes: the need for wider engagement. BMJ Qual Saf 2013;22(11):885–7. http://dx.doi.org/10.1136/bmjqs-2013-002444.
12. WHO. Task shifting: rational redistribution of tasks among health workforce teams: global recommendations and guidelines. Geneva (Switzerland): World Health Organization; 2008.
13. Farley LD, Mlandu N, Ndjeka N, et al. Nurse initiation and management of MDR-TB-HIV: lessons from operational research. 43rd Union conference on lung health. Kuala Lumpur, November 13–17, 2012.
14. Waga G, Mavoa H, Snowdon W, et al. Knowledge brokering between researchers and policy makers in Fiji to develop policies to reduce obesity: a process evaluation. Implement Sci 2013;8:74. http://dx.doi.org/10.1186/1748-5908-8-74.
15. Edwards R, Drumright L, Kiernan M, et al. Covering more territory to fight resistance: considering nurses' role in antimicrobial stewardship. J Infect Prev 2011; 12(1):6–10.

16. Duguid M, Cruickshank M, editors. Antimicrobial stewardship in Australian hospitals. Sydney (Australia): Australian Commission on Safety and Quality in Health Care; 2011. ISBN: 978-0-9870617-0-6.

17. Wertheim HF, Chandna A, Vu PD, et al. Providing impetus, tools, and guidance to strengthen national capacity for antimicrobial stewardship in Viet Nam. PLoS Med 2013;10:e1001429.

18. McNulty CA, Nichols T, French DP, et al. Expectations for consultations and antibiotics for respiratory tract infection in primary care: the RTI clinical iceberg. Br J Gen Pract 2013;63(612):e429–36. http://dx.doi.org/10.3399/bjgp13X669149.

19. Formoso G, Paltrinieri B, Marata AM, et al. LOCAAL Study Group. Feasibility and effectiveness of a low cost campaign on antibiotic prescribing in Italy: community level, controlled, non-randomised trial. BMJ 2013;347:f5391. http://dx.doi.org/10.1136/bmj.f5391.

20. Wutzke SE, Artist MA, Kehoe LA, et al. Evaluation of a national programme to reduce inappropriate use of antibiotics for upper respiratory tract infections: effects on consumer awareness, beliefs, attitudes and behavior in Australia. Health Promot Int 2007;22:53–64.

21. Available at: http://newsser.fda.moph.go.th/rumthai. Accessed October 30, 2013.

22. Charani E, Edwards R, Sevdalis N, et al. Behavior change strategies to influence antimicrobial prescribing in acute care: a systematic review [review]. Clin Infect Dis 2011;53(7):651–62. http://dx.doi.org/10.1093/cid/cir445.

23. Shekelle PG, Pronovost PJ, Wachter RM, et al. The top patient safety strategies that can be encouraged for adoption now. Ann Intern Med 2013;158(5 Pt 2): 365–8.

24. Charani E, Cooke J, Holmes A. Antibiotic stewardship programmes – what's missing? J Antimicrob Chemother 2010;65(11):2275–7.

25. Available at: http://healthmarketinnovations.org/program/accredited-drug-dispensing-outlets-addo. Accessed October 30, 2013.

26. Everybody's Business. Strengthening health systems to improve health outcomes. WHO's framework for action. Geneva (Switzerland): World Health Organisation; 2007. Available at: http://www.who.int/healthsystems. Accessed February 24, 2014.

Health Care Provider Education as a Tool to Enhance Antibiotic Stewardship Practices

Christopher A. Ohl, MD*, Vera P. Luther, MD

KEYWORDS

- Antibiotic stewardship • Antimicrobial stewardship
- Antibiotic stewardship education • Antibacterial agents • Antibiotic prescribing
- Prescribing • Health care personnel • Antibiotic resistance

KEY POINTS

- Education of health care providers is a key component of an antibiotic stewardship program.
- Antibiotic stewardship education for health care providers is recommended as a strategy to provide a foundation of knowledge and an environment that facilitates and supports optimal antibiotic prescribing.
- Antibiotic stewardship education should start early in the training of health care professionals and should include medical and other health care students, as well as practicing and training physicians and ancillary providers.
- The content of antibiotic stewardship education should include information on antibiotics and antibiotic resistance, teaching on core principles of diagnosis and management of infection, training on appropriate antibiotic prescribing, and coaching to improve communication skills.
- Passive antibiotic stewardship education techniques are modestly effective for increasing prescriber knowledge, whereas education using active techniques is more effective for changing prescribing behavior.
- Health care provider education on appropriate antibiotic prescribing has been shown to enhance other antibiotic stewardship interventions.

The authors have no conflicts of interest to disclose.
Section on Infectious Diseases, Center for Antimicrobial Utilization Stewardship and Epidemiology, Wake Forest School of Medicine, Wake Forest Baptist Medical Center, 100 Medical Center Boulevard, Winston-Salem, NC 27157, USA
* Corresponding author.
E-mail address: cohl@wakehealth.edu

Infect Dis Clin N Am 28 (2014) 177–193
http://dx.doi.org/10.1016/j.idc.2014.02.001
0891-5520/14/$ – see front matter © 2014 Elsevier Inc. All rights reserved.

INTRODUCTION

The overuse and inappropriate use of antibiotics are common worldwide and are associated with adverse drug reactions, *Clostridium difficile* infections, and increased health care costs.[1–3] Antibiotic misuse has been a major factor in the emergence of extensively multidrug-resistant pathogens over the last 2 decades.[4] Moreover, the number of new antibiotics recently approved or under development for treatment of these infections is alarmingly low, making current antibiotic drugs a precious commodity.[5] Antibiotic stewardship has been increasingly recognized as an important tool to combat antibiotic resistance, preserve current antibiotics, and improve patient care through the improvement of antibiotic prescribing at the level of the individual patient and on a larger scale for hospitals and health care systems.[4,6] Antibiotic stewardship practices include an array of potentially useful interventions of varying effectiveness for both inpatient and outpatient medicine. One of these practices is the provision of antibiotic stewardship education to health care provider students, clinical trainees, practicing clinicians, and ancillary personal, with the goal of improving antibiotic prescribing and use. In this review, the need and suggested audience for antibiotic stewardship education are highlighted, and effective education techniques are recommended for increasing knowledge of antibiotics and improving their use.

THE NEED FOR EDUCATION IN ANTIBIOTIC STEWARDSHIP

Education has been deemed to be the cornerstone of antibiotic stewardship. Usually, this education refers to improving the knowledge and prescribing behavior of current or future health care providers to reduce or improve their antibiotic use. Afterall, the success of a stewardship program depends on the attitude and action of individuals. Many have pointed out the need to expand antibiotic stewardship education to all of the relevant stakeholder groups, not just health care providers. These groups include patients, parents, children, governmental and regulatory authorities, and society as a whole.[7–10] Although important, education of health care consumers and other stakeholders in antibiotic stewardship falls outside the scope of this article, which focuses on education of health care providers.

The goal of education in antibiotic stewardship is to not only reduce the total use of antibiotics by an individual prescriber but to ensure that when an antibiotic is truly indicated, it is the right drug at the right dose, via the correct route, and for the proper duration. It can be reasonably assumed that a responsible clinician with proper clinical decision-making skills and sufficient knowledge of patient-specific clinical and microbiological data would use antibiotics wisely and correctly for every patient. However, up to 50% of antibiotic prescribing in both the inpatient and outpatient arena is unnecessary or suboptimal.[11–13] This actuality suggests that there are significant deficits in provider knowledge, skills, and data access. Serious deficits of knowledge in clinicians regarding appropriate antibiotic use have been recognized for some time by infectious diseases physicians, clinical microbiologists and pharmacists, medical professional societies, and public health entities.[4,6,9,14,15]

Recent studies have shed some light on prescribers' perceptions of their knowledge and clinical decision making in antibiotic use. Surveys of practicing physicians and teaching hospital faculty have shown that clinicians are aware of the relationship between antimicrobial use and resistance and that they believe that most physicians overprescribe antibiotics nationally and in their individual hospitals.[16,17] The survey respondents tended to believe that the problem of overprescription lay more with others than themselves, although most (>70%) would still like more knowledge about antibiotics and individual feedback on their antibiotic use.[16] Similar surveys of house staff physicians in training found comparable results, but in addition showed a surprising lack of knowledge in written tests of antibiotics and antibiotic use, which did not improve over the course of their training.[16,18] Regarding medical students, self-assessed perceptions and clinical vignette–based scores of antimicrobial use knowledge were evaluated by Abbo and colleagues[19] at 4 US medical schools. These investigators found a low mean knowledge score (51%). In addition, most student respondents believed their preparedness to be inadequate and would prefer more education on appropriate use of antibiotics during medical school. Similarly, medical students in Europe have also expressed a lack of confidence in their antibiotic knowledge and a desire for more antibiotic prescribing information.[20,21]

ON WHOM SHOULD ANTIBIOTIC STEWARDSHIP EDUCATION FOCUS?

To address health care provider knowledge deficits and a lack of clinical skills in antibiotic stewardship, professional societies and public health and governmental agencies worldwide have called for increased and improved education for practicing and training health care providers as well as for all medical and ancillary provider students (**Box 1**).[6,11,14,22] Such education initiatives in antibiotic stewardship have slowly arisen over the last decade and have primarily focused on practicing clinicians and, to some extent, on clinical pharmacists.

Antibiotic stewardship education should focus on improving antibiotic prescribing of practicing and training physicians, ancillary providers, and clinical pharmacists in both the outpatient and inpatient realms. However, in the United States, most professional society and public health educational efforts on the subject have, until recently, focused on training individuals on how to establish an inpatient antibiotic stewardship program rather than on training individual prescribers on how to improve their antibiotic use.[23] One prominent exception is outpatient antibiotic prescribing education for both health care providers and the general public, which has been available since 2003 from the Centers for Disease Control and Prevention's (CDC) *Get Smart about Antibiotics* campaign.[24] This successful program has recently been expanded to include education and materials on inpatient antibiotic stewardship. The European Union has had a more organized effort to promote antibiotic stewardship education for individual clinicians and the public, but for the most part, it has also focused on the outpatient antibiotic prescriber and consumer.[9,25] Nonetheless, as the number of hospitals and health care systems with active antibiotic stewardship programs

---

Box 1
Important targets for antibiotic stewardship education

Practicing clinicians in primary care and specialty medicine

    Physicians

    Physician assistants

    Nurse practitioners

    Clinical prescribing pharmacists

Clinical trainees: resident house staff and fellows

Medical and ancillary provider students

Nurses

Retail dispensing pharmacists

increases, the number that use antibiotic stewardship education interventions for health care providers also increases. In addition, these individual efforts in the inpatient domain are becoming more coordinated.

Antibiotic stewardship and appropriate antibiotic use education has long been neglected in medical schools worldwide. Little is known about the content, volume, and quality of medical school teaching in antibiotic resistance and stewardship, but most would agree that it is limited.[7–9] Recently, the importance of training medical students in antibiotic use has been recognized in the United States and Europe, and medical schools are beginning to include antibiotic stewardship principles in their curricula. It is now recommended that antibiotic resistance, pharmacology, and stewardship be incorporated into curriculum requirements for medical, ancillary provider, and nursing students.[9,20,22,26] Such education should begin with the basic science years and continue through the student's clinical training. Furthermore, the principles learned in medical school should be reinforced and expanded throughout postgraduate residency and fellowship training by means of formal training and mentorship.

In addition, other health care providers likely to benefit from antibiotic stewardship education include nurses and retail pharmacists, as well as students and residents in these professions.[27–29] Although education for these groups would likely not be as focused on prescribing and clinical decision making as it is for clinicians, it should cover basic principles of stewardship to optimize their participation in clinical care involving antibiotic use. Nursing education might be a particularly important strategy for improving antibiotic use in long-term care facilities, an important sector in intense need of antibiotic stewardship.

WHO SHOULD PROVIDE ANTIBIOTIC STEWARDSHIP EDUCATION?

The optimal provider of antibiotic stewardship education depends on the discipline, level of training, and in some instances, individual personality of the targeted learner. In addition, subject content or elements, the learning venue or environment, and specific educational strategy should be considered when choosing an educator. The education of practicing physicians in inpatient facilities or health care systems with a multidisciplinary antibiotic stewardship team is likely best provided by team members who are clinicians, clinical pharmacists, clinical microbiologists, and in some cases, hospital epidemiologists, with expertise in antibiotic therapy. Teachers for physicians in training might include academic clinicians or basic scientists as well. Other teachers of antibiotic stewardship for practicing providers might include presenters at specialty or professional meetings, practice colleagues or recognized thought leaders, ward or clinic pharmacists, or clinical outreach providers. These latter instructors or coaches might receive their training from their local or regional antibiotic stewardship teams or from various train the trainer sessions. In some medical centers, clinical pharmacists and outreach providers function as extensions of the antibiotic stewardship team, increasing its breadth and effectiveness. In some instances, regional public health entities, such as the California Antibiotic Stewardship Initiative, have provided teachers for education sessions on antibiotic stewardship in acute care medical facilities.[30]

For medical students, it is important that instructors in the relevant fields of microbiology, pharmacology, and infectious diseases, as well as from organ-based content courses, incorporate antibiotic stewardship information in their teaching materials. This teaching should include information on antibiotic resistance and its relationship to antibiotic use, fundamentals of infection diagnosis and management, appropriate antibiotic prescribing, and important adverse effects of inappropriate prescribing. Academic clinicians from all specialties who participate in preclinical and clinical training of medical and pharmacy students should be proficient in the guidelines and principles of antibiotic use and incorporate these in their large and small group learning sessions, inpatient ward rounds, and clinic-based teaching sessions. As with other topics in education, mentorship and teaching by example are fundamental to successful learning.

CONTENT OF ANTIBIOTIC STEWARDSHIP EDUCATION

Table 1 lists the main topics and corresponding principles, learning outcomes, and competencies that have been advocated for antibiotic stewardship education by the literature, medical professional societies, and public health, governmental, and educational entities. These topics include the fundamentals of antibiotic resistance and its relationship to antibiotic use, as well as aspects of clinical reasoning, diagnosis and management of infection, and specific behavioral changes to improve antibiotic prescribing. Although topic emphasis varies depending on the professional field and level of training of the learner, all are pertinent for the curriculum of health care professional students, as well as for training and practicing providers.

A solid foundation of knowledge in antibiotic resistance mechanisms and epidemiology, in addition to an understanding of the relationship of resistance to antibiotic use, is necessary for health care providers to understand the scope of the problem and the role that their own prescribing plays in putting their patients at risk. It is important that the assimilation of such knowledge begins early during medical school, is built on during clinical training, and is reinforced throughout postgraduate practice. Similarly, knowledge of the principles of diagnosis and management of infection are essential to the choice and appropriate use of antibiotics and should be taught through all stages of training. More specific subject matters, such as those listed as principles of infection management in **Table 1**, are important strategic concepts that are integral to the education curricula of resident and fellow trainees and practicing health care providers, but should be introduced during the clinical years of medical school training. Continuous training in patient communication skills is important for all students, trainees and medical providers, because these skills are often necessary when prescribing antibiotics, especially in outpatient settings.

Worldwide, there are few standardized national curricula in antibiotic stewardship for medical school or postgraduate training institutions. However, one such example is in Scotland, where the Doctors Online Training System (DOTS), a mandatory Web-based education resource for training physicians, has been used since 2009 for teaching appropriate antibiotic prescribing.[22] Similarly, in the United Kingdom, the *Prudent Antibiotic User (PAUSE)* Web site offers shared standardized teaching materials for prudent antibiotic prescribing for elective use during medical school training.[31] In the United States, an *Antimicrobial Stewardship Curriculum for Medical Students* has been devolved in conjunction with the CDC and the Association of American Medical Colleges.[26] This curriculum is freely available online for use by any undergraduate professional school or postgraduate training hospital and consists of 3 large group presentations, with corresponding examination questions, and 5 interactive small group activities, with a facilitator guide. These and other resources for education content are listed in **Box 2**.

To ensure uniform training and education for physicians in training, core education competencies in the various specialty topics are established. In the United Kingdom, such competences have been developed regarding principles of appropriate antibiotic prescribing, and physician trainees are evaluated on these competencies.[9]

Table 1
Content elements of antimicrobial stewardship education

Topic	Principles, Learning Outcomes, Competencies
Bacterial resistance	Genetics and mechanisms Extent and causes Epidemiology Relationship to antibiotic use
Antibiotics	Spectrum of activity Principles of empirical vs directed therapy Pharmacology and adverse effects, including risk of *Clostridium difficile* infection Drug purchasing and dispensing costs
Diagnosis of infection	Proper use and interpretation of bacterial Gram stain/culture, rapid and point-of-care tests, serology, and biomarkers of infection (eg, C-reactive protein, procalcitonin) Colonization vs infection Inflammation vs infection Establishment of standardized diagnosis criteria for specific infections (eg, community-acquired pneumonia, hospital-acquired pneumonia, cystitis, pyelonephritis) Define infection 3 ways Anatomy (infected organs and tissues) Microbiology Pathophysiology (eg, host factors, infection risk, secondary complications
Principles of infection management	Timely and appropriate initiation of antibiotics Promptly identify patients who require antibiotics Obtain cultures before starting antibiotics Do not give antibiotics with overlapping activity or combinations not supported by evidence or guidelines Determine and verify antibiotic allergies Consider local antibiotic susceptibility Specify expected duration of therapy based on evidence and national and hospital guidelines Appropriate administration (intravenous vs oral) Ensure antibiotics patient is receiving and start dates are visible at point of care Give antibiotics at the right dose and interval Stop or de-escalate therapy promptly based on the culture and sensitivity results or establishment of an alternative diagnosis (antibiotic time-out) Stop vancomycin when methicillin-resistant *Staphylococcus aureus* is not isolated on culture Stop inciting antibiotics when *Clostridium difficile* infection is diagnosed Reconcile and adjust antibiotics at all transitions and changes in patient's condition Monitor for toxicity reliably and adjust agent and dose promptly

(continued on next page)

Table 1
(continued)

Topic	Principles, Learning Outcomes, Competencies
Guidelines for diagnosis and management of specific infection	Specific instruction for each of these common infections using the principles outlined above
The big 4 in hospitalized patients	Use of national and local guidelines and public health guidance
Urinary tract infection and asymptomatic bacteriuria	
Community-acquired pneumonia	
Health care–acquired pneumonia	
Skin and soft tissue infection	
The big 4 in outpatients	
Sinusitis	
Acute bronchitis	
Pharyngitis	
Otitis media	
Prevention of infection	Principles and duration of surgical prophylaxis
	Hand hygiene
	Prudent use of catheters, devices
Communication skills	Discussion techniques with patients on why an antibiotic is not necessary and prudent antibiotic use

Adapted from Refs.[9,29,54]

Box 2
Online resources for education content for antibiotic stewardship

An Antibiotic Stewardship Curriculum for Medical Students

    http://www.wakehealth.edu/School/CAUSE/Get-Smart-About-Antibiotics.htm

Prudent Antibiotic User (*PAUSE*)

    http://www.pause-online.org.uk

Scottish Antimicrobial Prescribing Group

    http://www.scottishmedicines.org.uk/SAPG/Education/Education

Get Smart About Antibiotics (CDC)

    http://www.cdc.gov/getsmart/

    For health care professionals:

    http://www.cdc.gov/getsmart/specific-groups/hcp/index.html

Stanford Online course: *Antimicrobial Stewardship: Optimization of Antibiotic Practices* (CME)

    http://online.stanford.edu/course/antimicrobial-stewardship-optimization-antibiotic-practices

CDC and Institute for Healthcare Improvement *Antibiotic Stewardship Drivers and Change Package*

    http://www.cdc.gov/getsmart/healthcare/improve-efforts/driver-diagram/index.html

World Health Organization *Good Prescribing Guide*

    http://apps.who.int/medicinedocs/en/d/Jwhozip23e/

In the United States, such competences in antibiotic stewardship for trainees have not been established, other than broadly in the context of health care resource utilization.

EFFECTIVENESS OF EDUCATION TO CHANGE ANTIBIOTIC PRESCRIBING BEHAVIOR

The desired outcome of any antibiotic stewardship intervention, in either the inpatient or outpatient sector, is to change a clinician's attitude toward infection management and their antibiotic prescribing behavior. Antibiotic stewardship interventions involving education are no different. Thus, success as solely defined by a traditional measure of education effectiveness, improved or increased knowledge, is not sufficient. If education increases awareness or knowledge of antibiotic stewardship principles but does not effectively change prescribing behavior or attitudes, the desired outcome of education is not realized. The lessons learned with education in antibiotic stewardship are similar to those learned with education in clinical performance improvement, hospital infection prevention, and public health.[32,33] Improved clinician knowledge does not necessarily lead to improved clinician behavior.

For stewardship, the literature shows that some particular education techniques are effective mostly for increasing prescriber knowledge, whereas others additionally influence prescribing behavior.[9,11,33–35] In general, the former are passive techniques such as large and small group presentations, conferences, and guideline dissemination. The latter are more interactive or dynamic techniques, which include education that is associated with specific episodes of patient care, or combined with audit and feedback of a specific provider or practice's prescribing data. In addition to being more effective for changing prescribing behavior, active techniques tend to have results that are longer lasting than passive techniques.[33,35]

Results of effectiveness studies of education techniques in antibiotic stewardship among practicing clinicians tend to be similar to those evaluating continuing medical education in other disciplines.[36] Antibiotic stewardship guidelines for inpatient facilities from the Infectious Diseases Society of America (IDSA) and Society for Healthcare Epidemiology of America (SHEA), as well as many investigators with experience in antibiotic stewardship, advocate multifaceted education interventions combined with other effective antibiotic stewardship strategies.[9,11,23,33,34,37] Such strategies are believed to be more effective for improving antibiotic use if used together with education rather than if used alone. Moreover, there are limited data that the effects of interventions that combine antibiotic prescription preauthorization with passive or active education are more sustained then those that use preauthorization without education.[32] Although it is beneficial to include education activities in antibiotic stewardship interventions, a comprehensive approach might not always be necessary. A recent large meta-analysis[35] of antibiotic stewardship techniques and strategies found that complex multifaceted education interventions were not necessarily more effective than simpler methods.

Little is known about the effectiveness of education to improve the future pharmaceutical or antibiotic prescribing of medical students and clinical trainees.[38] A systematic review of the literature on education interventions to improve prescribing by these learners in 2009 found only 15 studies on the subject.[39] These were mostly small studies of students rather than trainees, subject to methodological flaws, and examined increased knowledge or improved prescribing for all drugs, not just antibiotics, in simulated rather than real patients. Only 1 intervention, the World Health Organization *Good Prescribing Guide*, had been tested in a variety of international settings across a range of students at different levels. Randomized trials of this intervention showed modest beneficial effects in preparing medical students for real-world pharmaceutical prescribing but did not examine whether graduates translated this knowledge into practice.[39]

There are also few studies of the effectiveness of structured education for clinical trainees. A prospective crossover study of medicine and family practice resident trainees in the United States showed that a 1-year interactive small group conference led by an antibiotic stewardship team significantly improved knowledge of proper antibiotic use.[40] These conferences used resident-supplied patient cases involving antibiotic management dilemmas from their own outpatient and inpatient clinical practice. However, this study did not examine whether this improved knowledge translated into better antibiotic prescribing practices. In Europe, early results from the 2009 implementation of the Scottish DOTS education resource do suggest that improved antibiotic prescribing and a reduction in *Clostridium difficile* infection are associated with clinical vignette–based training of house staff.[22] There is clearly a great need for more research to guide undergraduate and graduate medical education institutions on the most effective ways to teach appropriate antibiotic use.

BEHAVIORAL SCIENCE THEORY AND SOCIAL MARKETING

In acute care medical facilities, cultural, contextual, and behavioral determinants influence antibiotic prescribing as much, if not more than, anti-infective knowledge.[41,42] Behavioral science theories could be used to further understand the determinants of prescribing behavior to develop specific education interventions to improve antibiotic prescribing. Principles of behavioral and social science and commercial marketing have been used by public health in social marketing to change health behaviors to reduce the burden of disease on society. Such social marketing usually focuses on a target group with similar societal characteristics to develop research-driven behavior change interventions.[42] Examples of behavior changes associated with social marketing include smoking cessation and safe sex practices.

Although still in its infancy in acute care medical facilities, social marketing and associated personality profiling have the potential to assist antibiotic stewardship efforts.[43] Evidence from a few studies using these strategies indicates that the influence of senior colleagues on antibiotic prescribing is significant and that peer and opinion leader perceptions and behaviors have a greater influence on prescribing behavior when compared with local policies and guidelines.[42,44] This information could help direct academic detailing and educational outreach visits to optimize its effectiveness. A recent systematic review of studies in antibiotic prescribing behavior[42] found only a few studies that used behavioral sciences or social marketing in their methods or analysis. The investigators' conclusion was that despite qualitative evidence showing the impact of behavioral determinants and social norms on prescribing, these influences were not adequately assessed in research assessing interventions in antibiotic use. More research is needed on this important subject.

EDUCATION ACTIVITIES AND STRATEGIES TO INFLUENCE ANTIBIOTIC USE

Tables 2 and **3** list the types and characteristics of education activities and interventions that might be effective for improving antibiotic use and patient outcomes. These activities have been used and studied in various health care improvement initiatives, many of which focus on optimizing antibiotic use. Generally, these education activities can be classified into passive or active interventions, depending on their underlying nature and how they are implemented.[32] Another way of classifying these educational activities is whether they shape or change a health care provider's clinical behavior.[9] Regarding antibiotic stewardship, behavior shaping activities are ones that provide

Table 2
Types of education activities and interventions

Activities and Interventions	Intervention Type	Description
Didactic large group programs	Passive Shaping	Lectures and presentations with question answer sessions, continuing medical education
Interactive small group sessions	Passive or active Shaping	Interactive small group didactic workshops (eg, problem-based learning), real or hypothetical case presentation conferences with discussion, mortality and morbidity conference, role-playing sessions
e-Learning	Passive or active, depending on the module Shaping or changing	Interactive learning modules provided via computers, often Internet based
Distribution of informative printed material	Passive Shaping or changing	Printed guidelines, handouts, articles and reports, fact sheets, pocket-cards, newsletters by mail, fax, or during didactic education sessions
Reminders	Active Changing	Verbal, paper or computer-generated (eg, pop-up best practice advisories, sticky notes) prompts of the practitioner to provide a specific clinical intervention under defined clinical circumstances; often associated with the medical record
Local consensus processes or opinion/ thought leader development	Active Changing	Based on behavioral science and social marketing; advisory boards and committees/subcommittees, one-on-one discussion with providers for consensus building
Educational outreach	Active Changing	Academic detailing: one-on-one discussion by a trained professional with providers about their practice and prescribing behavior, including specific patient scenarios; includes dissemination of information on study outcomes, guidelines, and best medical practice(s)
Periodic retrospective audit and feedback	Active Changing	Periodic review of data on prescribing behavior of an individual provider or group practice, usually for a specific diagnosis or diagnosis group (eg, upper respiratory tract infections) and direct feedback to the provider(s), with recommendations for improved prescribing behavior
One-on-one patient-directed education	Active Changing	Direct instructional and education component of individual prospective audit with intervention and feedback (review and recommend change or postprescription review) or prescription/ order preauthorization intervention

Table 3
Efficacy and qualities of education activities and interventions

Activities and Interventions	Intervention Efficacy	Comments
Didactic large group programs	Low	More effective if identified by the learners as a serious clinical need Marginally effective for changing performance or behavior, although more effective for changing simple behaviors Need to be integrated with other interventions Useful for introducing background information and the need for a program; explaining interventions to prescribers; establishing buy-in Easy to integrate into conventional undergraduate medical and ancillary provider curricula Refs.[23,32–37]
Interactive small group sessions	Moderate	Few studies on impact on prescriber behavior or patient outcomes Effective learning technique for undergraduate medical and ancillary provider students, clinical trainees More resource intensive than large group learning Refs.[34–36]
e-Learning	Moderate	Not yet widely available for antibiotic stewardship training Effectiveness not well studied and extrapolated from other interactive learning methods One study in Europe using Internet-based training of providers in C-reactive protein and patient communication skills showed improved prescribing for acute respiratory tract infections Improved prescribing and *Clostridium difficile* infections seen in Scotland after launching an e-learning platform for antibiotic stewardship Potentially useful for practicing clinicians, but likely more valuable for students, residents, and fellows in clinical training Useful for outreach in rural areas Refs.[8,9,22,50]
Distribution of informative printed material	Low	A small beneficial effect on practice outcomes is seen when used alone; effect may be increased when used with other interventions Impact on patient outcomes unknown Refs.[9,11,34,35,46]
Reminders	Low to moderate	Printed reminder efficacy enhanced by providing space on the reminder for a response from the clinician and providing an explanation of the content/advice of the reminders In 1 systematic review, effect of computer-generated reminders was smaller than that expected from the implementation of computerized order entry and electronic medical record systems Many of the positive studies in antibiotic stewardship were multifaceted Refs.[34,35,51–53,55]

(continued on next page)

Table 3 (continued)		
Activities and Interventions	**Intervention Efficacy**	**Comments**
Local consensus processes or opinion/thought leader development	Low to moderate	Effects difficult to measure, may have greater effect than local policy and guidelines The more efficacious interventions use social marketing strategies Refs.[34,35,42,56]
Educational outreach	Moderate to high	The more efficacious outreach interventions use social marketing strategies Often performed in combination with other education activities Likely more effective than periodic retrospective audit and feedback An effective way to approach extreme prescribing outliers Can be difficult to make direct personal contact with prescribers in community hospitals/practices Labor intensive Refs.[34,35,42,56]
Periodic retrospective audit and feedback	Moderate	One of the most widely published activities for antibiotic stewardship, often in multifaceted approach Effectiveness increased when baseline performance is low and repeated periodic interventions are used Feedback should be both oral and written and include targets and an action plan Source of feedback important: better if respected clinician/colleague More research needed to compare methods of delivering feedback Refs.[34,35,48,49,57]
One-on-one patient-directed education	Moderate to high	No direct studies available; efficacy extrapolated from educational outreach

a knowledge base, background, conceptual framework, thought basis, and clinical attitude for antibiotic prescribing. Behavior changing activities, on the other hand, are ones that directly change or improve antibiotic prescribing and provide the clinician with tools for implementing change. Typically, education that shapes behavior takes place during undergraduate and early postgraduate training, whereas education that changes behavior is administered during more senior clinical training and clinical practice. However, there is, and should be, considerable overlap in the timeline when behavior shaping and changing education takes place, and such education should be continuous rather than interrupted.

As shown in **Table 3**, early studies of conventional passive education techniques, including large and small group presentations, showed marginal effectiveness in improving antibiotic use. This situation resulted in a relative de-emphasis of passive education as an intervention by many investigators and in the IDSA/SHEA antibiotic stewardship guidelines.[11,23,45] However, little is known about what synergistic effect passive education has with other interventions to improve antibiotic prescribing. Some data, including recent meta-analyses, have suggested that improved knowledge and acceptance of antibiotic stewardship principles through passive education increase the effectiveness of other interventions that improve antibiotic prescribing, in addition to the small effect that such education provides on its own.[23,32,34,35,46,47] Advantages of passive education are that it requires fewer resources and personnel than active education and is more easily integrated into the curricula of medical and ancillary provider schools. Many investigators recommend that at least some passive education elements should be included in the implementation of antibiotic steward-ship education.[35]

As opposed to passive education, active education interventions, as described in **Tables 2** and **3**, are considered to be more effective for changing antibiotic prescribing behavior. Active methods of learning are more easily used for education of practicing or training clinicians than for undergraduate learners, although students in clinical training are still likely to benefit. One element that many active interventions have in common is that they integrate specific patient cases into the education. Another shared component is the measurement and feedback of clinician prescribing data, with suggestions on improvement. Periodic retrospective audit and feedback, by which an antibiotic stewardship team member intermittently measures and evaluates antibiotic prescribing data over time for an individual provider or practice and subse-quently recommends to them areas for improvement, is an example of such active ed-ucation.[48,49] This activity is one of the most studied education interventions and is distinct from real-time postprescription review and feedback. Some active interven-tions, such as using local consensus processes, opinion and thought leader develop-ment, and educational outreach use behavior and social marketing techniques not unlike those used by pharmaceutical marketing and sales teams. A few active inter-ventions, particularly those that involve consensus building, educational outreach, and periodic retrospective audit and feedback, can sometimes be used to improve prescribing behavior in problematic outliers who significantly abuse antibiotics compared with their peers. Most active education interventions have an advantage in that they can more easily be adapted to local needs but also have a significant disadvantage in that they are resource and labor intensive. Also, they may require a fairly developed antibiotic stewardship team for implementation.

The core antibiotic stewardship program activities endorsed in the IDSA/SHEA guidelines are prospective audit and feedback and prescription preauthorization. Although technically not education interventions per se, both of these activities can provide excellent opportunities for teaching specific antibiotic stewardship principles to practicing clinicians, resident and fellow house staff, and occasionally medical stu-dents. For example, a real-time postprescription audit and feedback activity that con-tacts prescribers suggesting discontinuing antibiotics after 5 days of treatment of uncomplicated community-acquired pneumonia educates clinicians to de-escalate therapy without a feedback intervention. A phone call from a clinician to an infectious diseases clinician or clinical pharmacist to request prescription preauthorization for a restricted antibiotic is often a miniconsult, and the information imparted to the clinician on the approach to the patient's infection and therapy (whether or not approval is given) is one-on-one patient-centric education. Clinician education during these inter-actions could include information on general infection diagnosis and management, in addition to specific suggestions for therapeutic choice and duration. These patient-associated education interventions require stewardship team members to be well trained in anti-infective therapy. In addition, learning is generally enhanced if the mem-ber is a physician or clinical pharmacist who has earned the respect of the facility's medical staff.

Internet-based education, or e-learning, is a more recent intervention, which has yet to have an opportunity to generate a consensus of effectiveness data. However, early results are encouraging.[22,25,50] Advantages of e-learning include improved access to education (including in rural areas) and a potentially more interactive learning platform, which is theoretically more likely to modify prescribing behavior. In addition, there is less need for fiscal and labor resources once an e-learning platform is established; however, the labor costs of site maintenance and content update should be considered. Another potentially fertile resource for education that may improve prescribing behavior is modification of the electronic medical record for teaching and guiding patient care.[51] Although early studies of the impact on prescribing by incorporating best practice reminders into the electronic medical record have been disappointing,[52,53] the advantages of this technology, including clinical decision-making support, have yet to be fully developed.

THE FUTURE DIRECTION OF ANTIBIOTIC STEWARDSHIP EDUCATION

Formal antibiotic stewardship efforts including those using education are still in their infancy. Much needs to be done to develop and evaluate new and improved education techniques, curricular content, and interventions that not only increase knowledge and understanding of the subject but improve antibiotic prescribing and management. There is a clear need to develop standardized curricula in antibiotic stewardship for undergraduate medical education and postgraduate training. Such curricula should be widely incorporated into existing medical and ancillary provider schools, both in the preclinical and clinical years, and by academic medical centers with postgraduate trainees. Furthermore, postgraduate competencies should be developed and implemented that incorporate appropriate antibiotic prescribing and infection management. Postgraduate trainees should be held accountable to master these competencies.

For practicing physicians and other medical providers, continuing medical education provided by hospitals, regional and national professional medical societies, and public health entities should include antibiotic stewardship and its major principles and learning objectives in its content. In addition, antibiotic stewardship, infection diagnosis and management, infection prevention, and appropriate antibiotic prescribing should be included in professional board certification and recertification activities, including question-based knowledge modules and monitored practice improvement modules. Such a coordinated, multifaceted, continuous and longitudinal educational approach, in combination with other current and future antibiotic stewardship activities, holds much promise for improving antibiotic use, reducing adverse events caused by antibiotics, and potentially halting the spread of antibiotic resistance.

REFERENCES

1. Shehab N, Patel PR, Srinivasan A, et al. Emergency department visits for antibiotic-associated adverse events. Clin Infect Dis 2008;47(6):735–43.
2. Shaughnessy MK, Amundson WH, Kuskowski MA, et al. Unnecessary antimicrobial use in patients with current or recent Clostridium difficile infection. Infect Control Hosp Epidemiol 2013;34(2):109–16.
3. Beardsley JR, Williamson JC, Johnson JW, et al. Show me the money: long-term financial impact of an antimicrobial stewardship program. Infect Control Hosp Epidemiol 2012;33(4):398–400.
4. Centers for Disease Control and Prevention. Antibiotic resistance threats in the United States. 2013. Available at: http://www.cdc.gov/drugresistance/threat-report-2013/index.html. Accessed January 12, 2014.

5. Boucher HW, Talbot GH, Benjamin DK Jr, et al. 10 x '20 Progress–development of new drugs active against gram-negative bacilli: an update from the Infectious Diseases Society of America. Clin Infect Dis 2013;56(12):1685-94.

6. Society for Healthcare Epidemiology of America. Policy statement on antimicrobial stewardship by the Society for Healthcare Epidemiology of America (SHEA), the Infectious Diseases Society of America (IDSA), and the Pediatric Infectious Diseases Society (PIDS). Infect Control Hosp Epidemiol 2012;33(4):322-7.

7. Dryden MS, Cooke J, Davey P. Antibiotic stewardship–more education and regulation not more availability? J Antimicrob Chemother 2009;64(5):885-8.

8. McNulty CA, Cookson BD, Lewis MA. Education of healthcare professionals and the public. J Antimicrob Chemother 2012;67(Suppl 1):i11-8.

9. Pulcini C, Gyssens IC. How to educate prescribers in antimicrobial stewardship practices. Virulence 2013;4(2):192-202.

10. Stockley JM. European Antibiotic Awareness Day 2012: getting smart about antibiotics, a public-professional partnership. J Infect 2012;65(5):377-9.

11. Dellit TH, Owens RC, McGowan JE Jr, et al. Infectious Diseases Society of America and the Society for Healthcare Epidemiology of America guidelines for developing an institutional program to enhance antimicrobial stewardship. Clin Infect Dis 2007;44(2):159-77.

12. Shapiro DJ, Hicks LA, Pavia AT, et al. Antibiotic prescribing for adults in ambulatory care in the USA, 2007-09. J Antimicrob Chemother 2014;69(1):234-40.

13. Pulcini C, Cua E, Lieutier F, et al. Antibiotic misuse: a prospective clinical audit in a French university hospital. Eur J Clin Microbiol Infect Dis 2007;26(4):277-80.

14. World Health Organization. The evolving threat of antimicrobial resistance. Options for action. Available at: http://www.who.int/patientsafety/implementation/amr/publication/en/index.html. Accessed January 12, 2014.

15. Davey P, Hudson S, Ridgway G, et al. A survey of undergraduate and continuing medical education about antimicrobial chemotherapy in the United Kingdom. British Society of Antimicrobial Chemotherapy Working Party on Antimicrobial Use. Br J Clin Pharmacol 1993;36(6):511-9.

16. Abbo L, Sinkowitz-Cochran R, Smith L, et al. Faculty and resident physicians' attitudes, perceptions, and knowledge about antimicrobial use and resistance. Infect Control Hosp Epidemiol 2011;32(7):714-8.

17. Guerra CM, Pereira CA, Neves Neto AR, et al. Physicians' perceptions, beliefs, attitudes, and knowledge concerning antimicrobial resistance in a Brazilian teaching hospital. Infect Control Hosp Epidemiol 2007;28(12):1411-4.

18. Srinivasan A, Song X, Richards A, et al. A survey of knowledge, attitudes, and beliefs of house staff physicians from various specialties concerning antimicrobial use and resistance. Arch Intern Med 2004;164(13):1451-6.

19. Abbo LM, Cosgrove SE, Pottinger PS, et al. Medical students' perceptions and knowledge about antimicrobial stewardship: how are we educating our future prescribers? Clin Infect Dis 2013;57(5):631-8.

20. Davenport LA, Davey PG, Ker JS. An outcome-based approach for teaching prudent antimicrobial prescribing to undergraduate medical students: report of a Working Party of the British Society for Antimicrobial Chemotherapy. J Antimicrob Chemother 2005;56(1):196-203.

21. Dyar OJ, Pulcini C, Howard P, et al. European medical students: a first multicentre study of knowledge, attitudes and perceptions of antibiotic prescribing and antibiotic resistance. J Antimicrob Chemother 2014;69(3):842-6.

22. Nathwani D, Sneddon J, Malcolm W, et al. Scottish Antimicrobial Prescribing Group (SAPG): development and impact of the Scottish National Antimicrobial Stewardship Programme. Int J Antimicrob Agents 2011;38(1):16–26.
23. Tamma PD, Cosgrove SE. Antimicrobial stewardship. Infect Dis Clin North Am 2011;25(1):245–60.
24. Centers for Disease Control and Prevention. Get smart: know when antibiotics work. Available at: http://www.cdc.gov/getsmart/index.html. Accessed January 12, 2014.
25. McNulty CA. European Antibiotic Awareness Day 2012: general practitioners encouraged to TARGET antibiotics through guidance, education and tools. J Antimicrob Chemother 2012;67(11):2543–6.
26. Luther VP, Ohl CA, Hicks LA. Antimicrobial stewardship education for medical students. Clin Infect Dis 2013;57(9):1366.
27. Chahine EB, El-Lababidi RM, Sourial M. Engaging pharmacy students, residents, and fellows in antimicrobial stewardship. J Pharm Pract 2014;69(3):842–6.
28. Edwards R, Drumright L, Kiernan M, et al. Covering more territory to fight resistance: considering nurses' role in antimicrobial stewardship. J Infect Prev 2011; 12(1):6–10.
29. Crader MF. Development of antimicrobial competencies and training for staff hospital pharmacists. Hosp Pharm 2014;49(1):32–40.
30. Trivedi KK, Rosenberg J. The state of antimicrobial stewardship programs in California. Infect Control Hosp Epidemiol 2013;34(4):379–84.
31. British Society for Antimicrobial Chemotherapy, European Society of Clinical Microbiology and Infections Disease. Prudent antibiotic user (PAUSE). Available at: http://www.pause-online.org.uk. Accessed January 12, 2014.
32. Forsetlund L, Bjorndal A, Rashidian A, et al. Continuing education meetings and workshops: effects on professional practice and health care outcomes. Cochrane Database Syst Rev 2009;(2):CD003030.
33. Mazmanian PE, Davis DA, Galbraith R. Continuing medical education effect on clinical outcomes: effectiveness of continuing medical education: American College of Chest Physicians Evidence-Based Educational Guidelines. Chest 2009; 135(Suppl 3):49S–55S.
34. Cisneros JM, Cobo J, San JR, et al. Education on antibiotic use. Education systems and activities that work. Enferm Infecc Microbiol Clin 2013;31(Suppl 4): 31–7.
35. Davey P, Brown E, Charani E, et al. Interventions to improve antibiotic prescribing practices for hospital inpatients. Cochrane Database Syst Rev 2013;(4):CD003543.
36. Mazmanian PE, Davis DA. Continuing medical education and the physician as a learner: guide to the evidence. JAMA 2002;288(9):1057–60.
37. Ohl CA, Luther VP. Antimicrobial stewardship for inpatient facilities. J Hosp Med 2011;6(Suppl 1):S4–15.
38. Rubin P. A prescription for better prescribing: medical education is a continuum. BMJ 2006;333(7568):601.
39. Ross S, Loke YK. Do educational interventions improve prescribing by medical students and junior doctors? A systematic review. Br J Clin Pharmacol 2009; 67(6):662–70.
40. Luther VP, Petrocelli J, Beardsley J, et al. Effectiveness of a clinical reasoning curriculum to improve knowledge of appropriate antibiotic use. Presented at the 35th Annual Meeting of the Society for Medical Decision Making. Baltimore, MD, 22 October 2013.

41. Hulscher ME, Grol RP, van der Meer JW. Antibiotic prescribing in hospitals: a social and behavioural scientific approach. Lancet Infect Dis 2010;10(3):167–75.
42. Charani E, Edwards R, Sevdalis N, et al. Behavior change strategies to influence antimicrobial prescribing in acute care: a systematic review. Clin Infect Dis 2011;53(7):651–62.
43. Luther VP, Srnivasan A, High K, et al. Critical physician decision factors influencing appropriate antimicrobial prescribing in the hospitalized elderly. Presented at the Annual Meeting of the American Geriatrics Society. Washington, DC, 13 May 2011.
44. De Souza V, MacFarlane A, Murphy AW, et al. A qualitative study of factors influencing antimicrobial prescribing by non-consultant hospital doctors. J Antimicrob Chemother 2006;58(4):840–3.
45. Bantar C, Sartori B, Vesco E, et al. A hospitalwide intervention program to optimize the quality of antibiotic use: impact on prescribing practice, antibiotic consumption, cost savings, and bacterial resistance. Clin Infect Dis 2003;37(2):180–6.
46. Giguere A, Legare F, Grimshaw J, et al. Printed educational materials: effects on professional practice and healthcare outcomes. Cochrane Database Syst Rev 2012;(10):CD004398.
47. Kelley D, Aaronson P, Poon E, et al. Evaluation of an antimicrobial stewardship approach to minimize overuse of antibiotics in patients with asymptomatic bacteriuria. Infect Control Hosp Epidemiol 2014;35(2):193–5.
48. Chung GW, Wu JE, Yeo CL, et al. Antimicrobial stewardship: a review of prospective audit and feedback systems and an objective evaluation of outcomes. Virulence 2013;4(2):151–7.
49. Ivers N, Jamtvedt G, Flottorp S, et al. Audit and feedback: effects on professional practice and healthcare outcomes. Cochrane Database Syst Rev 2012;(6):CD000259.
50. Little P, Stuart B, Francis N, et al. Effects of internet-based training on antibiotic prescribing rates for acute respiratory-tract infections: a multinational, cluster, randomised, factorial, controlled trial. Lancet 2013;382(9899):1175–82.
51. Kullar R, Goff DA, Schulz LT, et al. The "epic" challenge of optimizing antimicrobial stewardship: the role of electronic medical records and technology. Clin Infect Dis 2013;57(7):1005–13.
52. Shojania KG, Jennings A, Mayhew A, et al. The effects of on-screen, point of care computer reminders on processes and outcomes of care. Cochrane Database Syst Rev 2009;(3):CD001096.
53. Shojania KG, Jennings A, Mayhew A, et al. Effect of point-of-care computer reminders on physician behaviour: a systematic review. CMAJ 2010;182(5): E216–25.
54. Centers for Disease Control and Prevention, Institute of Healthcare Improvement (IHI). Antibiotic Stewardship Drivers and Change Package. Available at: http://www.cdc.gov/getsmart/healthcare/improve-efforts/driver-diagram/index.html. Accessed January 12, 2014.
55. Arditi C, Rege-Walther M, Wyatt JC, et al. Computer-generated reminders delivered on paper to healthcare professionals; effects on professional practice and health care outcomes. Cochrane Database Syst Rev 2012;(12):CD001175.
56. Morris ZS, Clarkson PJ. Does social marketing provide a framework for changing healthcare practice? Health Policy 2009;91(2):135–41.
57. Gerber JS, Prasad PA, Fiks AG, et al. Effect of an outpatient antimicrobial stewardship intervention on broad-spectrum antibiotic prescribing by primary care pediatricians: a randomized trial. JAMA 2013;309(22):2345–52.

Antimicrobial Use Metrics and Benchmarking to Improve Stewardship Outcomes
Methodology, Opportunities, and Challenges

Omar M. Ibrahim, PhD[a], Ron E. Polk, PharmD[b],*

KEYWORDS

- Antibiotic use • Antibiotic metrics • Antibiotic resistance • Benchmarking
- Antibiotic stewardship • Antibiotic epidemiology

KEY POINTS

- Professional organizations recommend that antimicrobial stewardship programs measure their antimicrobial drug use and the clinical outcomes of interventions that change drug use.
- The recommended metric to quantify inpatient antimicrobial drug use in the United States is days of therapy per 1000 patient-days. Additional metrics are being evaluated.
- Benchmarking risk adjusted antibiotic use across multiple hospitals is possible; research is needed to determine if stewardship programs will use the information to develop interventions resulting in improved antibiotic use.
- Stewardship interventions have historically focused on process measures and economic savings; research of the effectiveness of stewardship on clinical outcomes, including bacterial resistance, is needed to justify long-term viability.

INTRODUCTION: NATURE OF THE PROBLEM

All antimicrobial stewardship programs (ASPs) have a common goal: to improve the quality of antibiotic prescribing. It follows that a successful ASP must be able to accomplish 2 tasks: (1) measure antimicrobial usage to know if an intervention was effective in changing antimicrobial use and (2) measure an outcome related to the

Funding Support: The authors have nothing to disclose.
Conflicts of Interest: The authors have nothing to disclose.
[a] Department of Pharmaceutical Outcomes and Policy, College of Pharmacy, University of Florida, 1225 Center Drive, Gainesville, FL 32611, USA; [b] Department of Pharmacotherapy and Outcomes Science, School of Pharmacy, Virginia Commonwealth University/Medical College of Virginia Campus, 410 North 12th Street, Richmond, VA 23298, USA
* Corresponding author.
E-mail address: rpolk@vcu.edu

Infect Dis Clin N Am 28 (2014) 195–214
http://dx.doi.org/10.1016/j.idc.2014.01.006
0891-5520/14/$ – see front matter © 2014 Elsevier Inc. All rights reserved.

change in use. Nearly all position papers from professional organizations and expert commentaries support these 2 tasks (**Box 1**).

Outcomes of ASPs historically focused on reducing costs of antimicrobial therapy,[11] and this focus continues for many programs.[12–14] Recent attempts to refocus stewardship outcomes have stressed clinical measures, including reductions in rates of bacterial resistance and *Clostridium difficile* infection (CDI) (see **Box 1**). Two recent reviews discussed the importance of linking ASP activities to clinical outcomes, including bacterial resistance.[15,16] As John McGowan, a stewardship pioneer, emphasized, "Measurements of the success of these programs have focused primarily on process measures. However, evaluation of outcome measures will be needed to ensure sustainability of these efforts."[16] In this review, measurement of aggregate

---

Box 1
Recommendations to measure antimicrobial use and the consequences of an intervention

- ASPs "must establish process and outcome measures to determine the impact of antimicrobial stewardship on antimicrobial use and resistance patterns."[1]

- "Research on Antimicrobial Stewardship Is Needed. Two primary issues of equal importance must be considered: (1) the benchmarking of antimicrobial use within and between institutions, and the most effective and efficient interventions to optimize these measures; and (2) the development of clear, well-defined, and validated process and outcome measures that may be utilized to assess the clinical impact of stewardship efforts."[2]

- "Intervention-specific outcome data should be collected after the intervention is implemented to demonstrate the continued benefit of the program. Outcomes can include costs, days on antibiotics, changes in prescription practices of a specific antibiotic, trends in MDROs or *Clostridium difficile*."[3]

- "Although the aim of [ASPs] has traditionally been to guide antimicrobial usage, the guidelines emphasize that this is a proxy (process variable) for the ultimate goal of controlling antimicrobial resistance and improving patient outcomes (outcome variables). Proper measurement of these variables is essential to ascertain the effectiveness of an antimicrobial stewardship program."[4]

- "C.2.a. [The] Facility has a multidisciplinary process in place to review antimicrobial utilization, local susceptibility patterns, and antimicrobial agents in the formulary *and* there is evidence that the process is followed."[5]

- "When asked to rank the most important final indicators with respect to both quality improvement and public reporting purposes...all respondents ranked [antibiotic] days of therapy and readmission rates among the most important areas on which to focus, irrespective of feasibility."[6]

- "The change in antimicrobial usage is the most common outcome measured in studies of stewardship programs. Common outcome variables related to antimicrobial usage include quantity of total antimicrobial use, quantity of targeted antimicrobial use, duration of therapy, percentage of oral versus intravenous drug administration, and antimicrobial drug expenditures."[7]

- "Stewardship metrics: Measuring outcomes. Documentation of fiscal and clinical outcomes is required for sustainability of most antimicrobial stewardship programs."[8]

- "Use of antibiotics as quality metrics often measures process instead of outcome, but remain important benchmarks for hospitals to use in national benchmarks. Antibiotic stewardship programs must monitor all aspects of antibiotic use, not just total consumption or costs"[9]

- "...antibiotic use data will have to be linked with an intervention strategy to reduce overuse and misuse of antibiotics."[10]

antimicrobial use in adult inpatients, the application to interhospital comparisons (benchmarking), and the role of these activities on clinical outcomes are discussed.

Essential Participants

ASPs have been described for more than 3 decades.[7] However, the recent surge in antimicrobial resistance rates and emergence of antibiotic-resistant superbugs, coupled with the paucity of new and novel antimicrobials, highlight the need for more comprehensive, coordinated, multifaceted, and interdisciplinary programs.[17-20] ASPs commonly include physicians, pharmacists, information technologists, clinical microbiologists, and infection control practitioners and vary in personnel depending on available resources. As discussed later, we believe that an essential participant in ASP efforts for programs with sufficient resources is a data analyst familiar with outcomes research.

MANAGEMENT STRATEGIES
Process Versus Outcomes

Box 1 includes frequent reference to elements from the Donabedian model of health care quality measurements, specifically the terms process and outcomes measures.[21] Wikipedia states, "...the Donabedian Model continues to be the dominant paradigm for assessing the quality of health care. According to the model, information about quality of care can be drawn from 3 categories: structure, process, and outcomes."[21] Applying this model to ASPs, structure is the presence or absence of an ASP, process refers to an ASP intervention to improve antibiotic use, and outcome refers to economic or clinical outcomes from the intervention. In the Donabedian model, "Outcomes [measures] are sometimes seen as the most important indicators of quality because improving patient health status is the primary goal of healthcare. However, accurately measuring outcomes that can be attributed exclusively to healthcare is very difficult. Drawing connections between process and outcomes often requires large sample sizes, adjustments by case mix, and long-term follow up as outcomes may take considerable time to become observable."[21] The implication for stewardship is that linking an ASP intervention to improve drug use and a subsequent change in clinical outcomes, such as improved response to therapy or changes in bacterial resistance, is more challenging than showing that an intervention was successful in only changing antibiotic use (a process measure).

INTERVENTIONS TO REDUCE ANTIMICROBIAL USE

Although measurement of antibiotic use is a process measure, antibiotics are unlike other drugs because excessive use compromises their usefulness; improved antibiotic use after an ASP intervention remains a critical metric to ensure future availability of this valuable medical resource (see **Box 1**). Because all ASPs attempt to change antibiotic use, the common measures of antimicrobial use are summarized first, followed by the role of benchmarking as a tool to improve use.

Antimicrobial Use Measures

Table 1 presents a summary of the aggregate antimicrobial use measures discussed in this subsection and their application. Measurement of aggregate antimicrobial use is only one of many ways to address the relationship of antibiotic consumption to outcome measures.[15] For example, case control studies link antimicrobial use at the individual patient level to clinical outcomes such as culture and susceptibility data.[10,15] These data will soon be available to ASPs in real time as the US health

Table 1

A summary of the common measures of antimicrobial use. These hypothetical calculations are based on a ward with 10 adult admissions in a month period with an average length of stay of 10 days. Eight patients received antimicrobial therapy for a mild to moderate severity community-acquired intra-abdominal infection, of whom 4 received monotherapy with intravenous (IV) ertapenem 1 g/d for 10 days (ward total = 40 g) and 4 received combination therapy (initiated concurrently) with ertapenem IV 1 g/d for 8 days (ward total = 32 g) and metronidazole IV 1.5 g/d for 7 days (ward total = 42 g). The remaining 2 patients did not receive antimicrobial therapy

Measure	Calculation	Relative Advantages	Relative Disadvantages	How ASPs Can Use the Measure
DOT/1000 PD	Total number of DOT = 40 d ertapenem (monotherapy patients) + 28 d ertapenem + 32 d metronidazole + 32 d ertapenem (combination therapy patients) = 100 DOT Total number of PD = number of admissions (10 admissions)* average LOS (10 d/admission) = 100 PD (100 DOT/100 PD)*1000 = 1000 DOT/1000 PD	DOT Not affected by changes in WHO reference DDDs, discrepancies between DDD and the prescribed dose or formulary mix Measures pediatric use The current US standard metric PD Incorporates LOS in the antimicrobial use measure, a form (although insufficient) of risk adjustment	DOT Does not measure dosage May underestimate exposure in renal impairment Does not estimate the duration of therapy Requires patient-level data Hospitals may measure use from different sources, such as billing or drug administration records complicating benchmarking comparisons US comparisons with countries using DDD methods problematic PD Inflates apparent use if LOS declines over time Requires knowledge of number of treated patients to properly interpret	DOT is replacing DDD as the primary antimicrobial use metric in the United States. Can be used to monitor impact of interventions on overall use and, after risk adjustment, to facilitate interhospital comparisons Redundant anaerobic coverage of ertapenem and metronidazole (second column) means an intervention to prevent metronidazole therapy reduces the total DOT measure from 100 to 68
DOT/1000 admissions	(100 DOT/10 admissions)* 1000 = 10,000 DOT/1000 admissions	Admissions in the denominator Not a function of LOS May correlate better than PD with bacterial resistance (requires additional study)	Admissions in the denominator Does not consider LOS; must be risk adjusted before used for benchmarking An unfamiliar metric for most hospitals with little validation at this time	Recommended as a secondary measure in addition to DOT/1000PD

Measure	Example calculation	Advantages	Limitations	Interpretation
DDD/1000PD	WHO standard reference values, IV ertapenem DDD = 1 g, IV metronidazole DDD = 1.5 g. Number of DDDs IV ertapenem = 40 g/1 g (monotherapy) + 32 g/1 g (combination therapy) = 72 DDDs, IV metronidazole = 42 g/1.5 g = 28 DDDs. Total number of DDDs = 1000 DDDs/1000 PD	Standardized comparisons of antimicrobial use between hospitals and countries. Easily calculated. Does not require patient-level data. May facilitate cost calculations because grams are measured	Overestimates or underestimates DOT when reference DDD is different from administered dose. Not applicable to pediatrics. Underestimates exposure in renal impairment (like DOT). Hospitals may measure use from different sources, such as purchase or drug administration records, which may complicate interhospital comparisons. WHO updates DDD reference values periodically complicating assessment of use over time	DDD may be used to benchmark intrahospital use over time if there are no changes in the WHO reference values or the antimicrobial formulary of the hospital. DDD can compare use of a specific antimicrobial between hospitals but is not well suited to benchmarking
LOT/discharge or admission (include only patients who received antimicrobial therapy)	Total number of LOT (d) = 40 d of ertapenem (monotherapy patients) + 28 d of both metronidazole and ertapenem (treatment days 1–7 in combination therapy patients) + 4 d of ertapenem (treatment day 8 in combination therapy patients) = 72 d. Average LOT = 72 d/8 treated patients = 9 d per treated patient	Provides an aggregate-level estimate of the average duration of therapy among patients who received antibiotics. Most useful when limited to specific clinical services or hospital units. Dose-independent (can be used in pediatrics)	Not normalized for LOS, should be risk adjusted for SOI or case mix before used for benchmarking. Unlike DOT, LOT cannot be used to compare use of specific drugs. Cannot discriminate between treatment periods (eg, cannot discriminate between 1 treatment period for 10 consecutive d vs 2 treatment periods of 5 d each). Does not reflect combination therapy or administered dosage. Patient-level data are needed for its calculation	A tertiary measure. ASPs can use this measure to identify units or service lines in which duration of therapy is excessive compared with other hospitals treating similar patients or to national standards. In the example provided, the average LOT of 9 d for treating patients with a mild to moderate community-acquired intra-abdominal infection is longer than the 4–7 d recommended by national treatment guidelines[22], a potential target for ASP intervention

(continued on next page)

Table 1
(continued)

Measure	Calculation	Relative Advantages	Relative Disadvantages	How ASPs Can Use the Measure
LOT/1000 PD	(72 d/100 PD)*1000 = 720 LOT/1000 PD	Can be calculated for all admissions in a unit or service line providing a measure of the intensity of antimicrobial use. Normalized for LOS making it possibly useful for benchmarking purposes	A proportion that does not estimate the duration of therapy. Patient-level data are needed for its calculation	A tertiary measure. ASPs can use this measure in conjunction with the DOT/LOT ratio and the proportion of treated patients (below) to identify whether high usage in units or service lines with high DOT/1000 PD is driven by potentially excessive durations of therapy, combination of therapy, a high proportion of treated patients, or a combination of these measures
DOT/LOT ratio	100 d/72 d = 1.40	Provides a measure for combination therapy at the aggregate level	Does not measure the proportion of patients who receive combination therapy. Patient-level data are needed for its calculation	A tertiary measure. ASPs may use this measure to identify potentially unnecessary combination antimicrobial drug use in specific units or service lines
Proportion receiving antimicrobial therapy	8 treated patients/10 admissions = 0.8	Provides another dimension of antimicrobial use that can be targeted by ASPs	Risk adjustment must ensure that groups being compared are similar in number and severity of infections	ASPs can use this measure to identify potentially unnecessary antimicrobial treatment in units or service lines with a higher proportion of treated patients compared with the benchmark, such as treatment of colonization (eg, asymptomatic bacteriuria) in patients with a Foley catheter

Abbreviations: DDD, defined daily dose; DOT, days of therapy; IV, intravenous; LOS, length of stay; LOT, length of therapy; PD, patient-days; SOI, severity of illness; WHO, World Health Organization.

care system implements electronic medical records (EMRs).[23] As reviewed by Jacob and Gaynes, "Studies using both approaches [aggregate and patient-level measures of use] are needed to create a better understanding of the efficacy of ASPs."[9]

Numerator Metric for Aggregate Use

Aggregate antimicrobial use is usually expressed as a rate at which the use metric (numerator) is normalized for hospital census (denominator). The 2 common metrics for measuring aggregate antimicrobial use are the defined daily dose (DDD) and the days of therapy (DOT).[9,10,15] The goal of the DDD metric is to estimate the DOT, often using antibiotic purchase data which are readily available. DDD is the measure promoted by the World Health Organization,[24] and it is the most widely used metric in Europe where electronic capture of billing, dispensing, or bar code administration data are generally unavailable.[25] In a 2011 survey of California hospitals, of 63 hospitals that measured their antimicrobial consumption (among 223 survey respondents), 11 used DDD and 8 used DOT; the remaining 44 hospitals did not respond.[26] If these data are representative of US acute care hospitals, measurement of antimicrobial use seems to be uncommon and of mixed methodology.

Because of limitations of the DDD method (see **Table 1** and later discussion),[27] many US hospitals measure the DOT directly from billing or dispensing data, and increasingly from bar code administration data.[28,29] Epic (Verona, WI; http://www.epic.com/), the largest vendor of EMR technology in the United States, uses DOT to measure use,[23] as does the Centers for Disease Control and Prevention (CDC) National Healthcare Safety Network (NHSN) (DOT is called *antimicrobial days* by NHSN).[30,31] An additional metric is the length of therapy (LOT, in days) and is the duration of therapy irrespective of the number of antimicrobials administered each day.[32] LOT can be used with other complementary measures, including the DOT/LOT ratio, to estimate the average number of antimicrobials administered.[32] The proportion of patients who receive antimicrobial therapy compared with a group of similar patients at a comparable institution may provide ASPs with another useful measure.[32]

Denominator Metric for Aggregate Use

The numerator of the aggregate antimicrobial use measure is usually divided by a measure of hospital occupancy such as the total number of patient-days (PD) or number of admissions, normalized to 100 or 1000 patients. PDs is the product of the number of admitted patients and the mean length of stay (LOS). The antimicrobial use option of the CDC's NHSN uses the denominator metric *days present*. Days present is defined as the total days that any patient received care in a specific patient-care location for any time during a day (a patient transferred from one location to another would count as a day present in each location).[30,31] When applied to hospital-wide antibiotic use, days present is equivalent to PDs.

In any hospital, the mean LOS may decrease over time as patients are discharged earlier, thereby decreasing PDs and increasing the apparent antibiotic use. Consequently, the number of admissions has been proposed as an alternative measure for tracking use trends over time,[33,34] and 1 study[35] found admissions to be superior to PDs for assessing the association between antimicrobial use and resistance. Consequently, hospitals may wish to express antimicrobial use normalized to 1000 admissions as a secondary measure, a strategy also recommended by the NHSN.[30]

The standard measure of aggregate antimicrobial use in US inpatient facilities is DOT/1000PD; improved measures may be forthcoming as this research progresses.

Platt's comment regarding benchmarking of health care–associated infections is also relevant to measurement of antimicrobial use: "It is widely believed that you cannot manage what you cannot measure. It is also true that you cannot measure what you cannot define."[36]

Benchmarking Antimicrobial Use

The Infectious Diseases Society of America and Society for Healthcare Epidemiology of America 2007 guidelines for ASPs[1] and other US policy statements and commentaries[2,3,9,30,31] recommend that hospitals benchmark their antimicrobial use for interhospital comparisons (see **Box 1**), after risk adjustment for differences in patient mix (see later discussion). The goal of benchmarking is to identify hospitals or clinical services within hospitals, in which observed antimicrobial use deviates significantly from that predicted (ie, low and high outliers). This strategy should allow ASPs to perform a drug utilization evaluation (DUE) in an area of high usage and identify intervention strategies. Such strategies may include reducing the duration of therapy to more closely match the benchmark, a reduction in the proportion of patients who receive antimicrobial therapy, or a reduction in the use of combination therapies (see **Table 1**). Conversely, the DUE may reveal unusual patterns of bacterial resistance or a mean severity of illness (SOI) in the patient population greater than the benchmark; this information may justify a different pattern or volume of use than the benchmark.

Risk adjustment is an integral part of benchmarking of health care outcomes and public reporting, because underlying disease(s) and comorbidities of the patient population (patient mix) are major determinants of using hospital resources, including antimicrobial consumption.[1,10,32,35] To show the need for risk adjustment, **Fig. 1** summarizes hospital-wide adult inpatient antibacterial and antifungal drug use during 2012 in a consortium of 97 US academic medical center hospitals that participate in the University HealthSystem Consortium (http://www.uhc.edu/). These data are aggregated from patient-level billing records, as previously described.[32] Antibacterial and antifungal drug use in hospitals 5 and 85 is exceptionally high. However, both hospitals serve almost exclusively an oncology patient population, and the unadjusted raw usage data in **Fig. 1** cannot be fairly compared with other hospitals. Consequently, interhospital comparisons of antibacterial and antifungal drug use must first be corrected for differences in patient mix (or SOI) for comparisons to be valid. We have recently described a method for risk adjusting antimicrobial use based on differences in patient mix across the academic medical center hospitals in **Fig. 1**.[32,37]

Alternative strategies to facility-wide benchmarking are becoming available. For example, the NHSN recommends that hospitals quantify antibiotic use in selected patient care areas, such as intensive care units, in addition to facility-wide measures.[30,31] When fully implemented, the NHSN program will add an important new dimension to the ability of a participating hospital to track use over time and to benchmark use across participating hospitals in multiple inpatient care units. Furthermore, benchmarking within selected inpatient units in which antibiotic use is high and in which resistance is often more common may facilitate ASP interventions with the greatest potential to improve patient care. A hospital ASP may also wish to benchmark their antimicrobial use within a given patient population against national standards, such as the timing of surgical prophylaxis or the timing of the first antimicrobial dose in the immunocompromised patient population.[37] Additional strategies and outcome evaluations are needed to fully realize the potential of benchmarking.

Risk adjustments methods that have been applied to benchmark antimicrobial use include regression modeling,[38–41] indirect standardization,[32,42] and direct standardization.[43] The details of these investigations have been reviewed elsewhere.[37] The

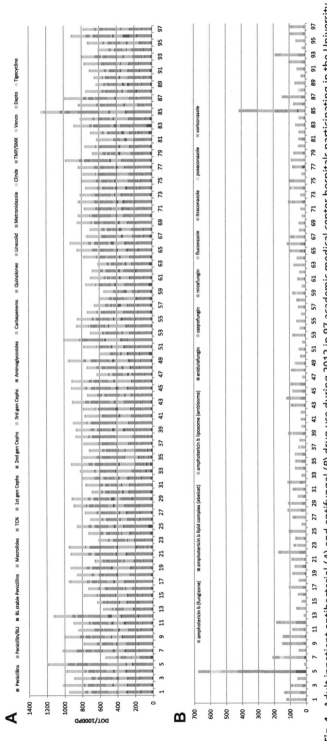

Fig. 1. Adult inpatient antibacterial (*A*) and antifungal (*B*) drug use during 2012 in 97 academic medical center hospitals participating in the University HealthSystem Consortium (http://www.uhc.edu/). These data represent raw drug usage figures that require risk adjustment to make them comparable across hospitals. See **Fig. 2** for an example of a risk adjusted interpretation of antibacterial drug use for 1 hospital. BL, beta-lactam; BLI, beta-lactamase inhibitor; DOT, days of therapy; PD, patient-days; TCN, tetracycline; TMP/SMX, trimethoprim/sulfamethoxazole.

following discussion reviews some of the methodological issues, common pitfalls, and areas in which additional work is needed.

Risk Adjustment Methods: Regression Analysis

Regression model analysis is the most widely used risk adjustment procedure and has been used to benchmark antimicrobial use.[38–41] The strategy to develop the regression model and its application to risk adjust antimicrobial drug use are summarized as follows.

- Conduct univariable analysis to identify a set of potential predictors of antimicrobial drug use, such as the number of infections, number of patients at risk (eg, transplants), Case Mix Index (CMI) for the facility or hospital unit, and so forth
- Apply a model selection procedure to identify a best subset of predictors of antimicrobial use from the set identified in the univariable analysis
- Fit the regression model using the subset of predictors identified
- Use the estimated regression equation to derive the predicted antimicrobial use for each unit of analysis (eg, hospital)
- Construct a prediction interval (typically a 95% or 90% interval) around each predicted value
- Classify each observation as a high outlier, low outlier, or an inlier depending on whether its observed value falls higher than the upper bound, lower than the lower bound, or within the 2 bounds of the prediction interval, respectively

AREAS IN WHICH MORE WORK IS NEEDED

- Most multivariable regression models applied to benchmarking were developed in Europe, where DDD/1000PDs was the outcome metric.[39,41] Although the DDD methodology does measure antibiotic use in a facility, it is severely compromised by a major confounder: the DDD value for total antibiotic use is also affected by the hospital's formulary composition.[37] Consequently, the DOT/1000 PD metric is becoming the standard measure for quantifying aggregate antimicrobial use in the United States, especially when used for benchmarking.
- Additional measures may improve on the DOT method as research progresses in this field. Traditional predictors of antimicrobial use, such as the number of infections and surgeries, generally explain only a modest percentage of the variability in use.[40,43,44] Identifying optimal predictors may also depend on the outcome metric. For example, we found that traditional predictors explained a higher percentage of the variability ($\approx$64%) when the DOT was normalized to 1000 discharges, versus 31% of the variability explained when normalized to PDs.[43] These observations require confirmation, and additional work may improve on identifying predictors in regression models.
- Benchmarking models should adjust for predictors of antimicrobial use that are considered nonmodifiable from the hospital or ASP perspective. Nonmodifiable predictors include hospital characteristics that are beyond the control of the hospital, such as the CMI and patient mix. We expect hospitals with a greater CMI for example, to use more antimicrobial drugs, and we include this in the model to predict use. On the other hand, presence or absence of an ASP is a modifiable variable and would not be included as a predictor. If our model finds that hospitals that tend to use fewer antimicrobials, after adjustment for nonmodifiable variables, also tend to be those with an ASP, we can then test if presence of an ASP is significantly associated with lower use.

- Sample size is a concern in regression modeling, especially when the analysis is performed at the aggregate hospital or unit level. One rule of thumb is that 10 observations (eg, hospitals or intensive care units) are needed for each predictor in the model (eg, number of infections).[45] Consequently, many hospitals or other units of analysis are needed to identify all important predictors.
- The traditional stepwise model selection procedures, including forward selection, backward elimination, and stepwise regression, continue to be widely used, despite recognized shortcomings.[46,47] Some alternative selection procedures include all-possible-subsets regression, least angle regression,[48] and the least absolute shrinkage and selection operator.[49] Although these procedures may be generally superior to the traditional stepwise selection procedures, all automated selection procedures have intrinsic limitations. Their major limitation lies in that there is no guarantee that they select the best model and that they generally do not perform well in the presence of a high degree of multicollinearity (the situation in which 2 or more predictor variables are highly correlated). For example, the hospital CMI, the number of transplants, and the number of infections are all likely to be related; including all 3 in an automated selection procedure to predict antibiotic use may lead to a multicollinearity problem, which is manifested by selection of predictors that are arbitrary and of low validity.
- An important limitation of classic regression models, including linear and logistic regression, is that the parameter estimates and the predictive capabilities of the model are sensitive to outliers. This sensitivity creates a paradoxic situation when using these models for benchmarking, because the identification of outliers is a pivotal procedure in benchmarking protocols. Moreover, an outlier observation inflates the estimated variance of the model, leading to a larger standard error and consequently, a wider confidence interval around the predicted value for that observation. Consequently, including an outlier observation in the model may make the model less likely to identify it as an outlier and, although all observations are used to develop the model, the procedure of determining the outlier status should be carried out using a model fitted without the observation in question. This strategy is especially recommended when the sample size is small. Robust regression is an alternative to classic linear regression, which is less sensitive to outliers and influential observations.[50]

Risk Adjustment Methods: Standardization

Standardization of rates is commonly used in epidemiology for benchmarking health care outcomes and hospital performance.[51–53] The 2 main standardization techniques are direct and indirect standardization; both have been applied to benchmark adult antibacterial drug use.[32,43] The procedure for their application to risk adjust antimicrobial drug use is summarized in **Box 2**.

Indirect standardization can also be used with regression modeling when patient-level data are available, giving it the flexibility of regression analysis by adjusting for many confounders.[51] Kanerva and colleagues[42] used this approach to benchmark antibiotic use in a sample of Finnish hospitals. However, even when risk adjusted, the direct comparison of indirectly standardized rates from either the regression-based approach or the stratification-based approach (see **Box 2**) may be inappropriate, unless there is considerable overlap in the distribution of the confounders between the hospitals.[51,54]

Using indirect standardization, we risk adjusted adult inpatient antibacterial use during 2009 in 70 academic medical center hospitals.[32,37] Graphical reports allowed an ASP to compare their observed hospital-wide antibacterial drug use to the risk

---

Box 2
General procedure for the application of direct and indirect standardization to benchmark antimicrobial drug use

- Patients are stratified into mutually exclusive strata, such as orthopedics or psychiatry such that the patient mix is expected to be homogenous and antimicrobial use is expected to be similar across hospitals within each stratum.

- The number of patients and the number of DOTs (or DDDs or LOT) are determined for each stratum within each hospital and are used to calculate the stratum-specific antimicrobial use rates (eg, DOT/discharge and DOT/1000PD).

- The data from all study hospitals is commonly pooled to create the reference population. The stratum-specific rates in the reference population can either be averages or weighted averages of the stratum-specific rates of the study hospitals.

- The direct standardization procedure is carried out by multiplying the stratum-specific antimicrobial use rate within each study hospital by the number of patients in the corresponding stratum of the reference population. This procedure generates an expected number of DOTs in each stratum, which are then summed across all strata to obtain the total expected number of DOTs. Total DOTs is divided by the total number of patients in the reference population to derive a directly standardized rate for each hospital. The directly standardized rates can then be directly compared between the study hospitals.

- The indirect standardization procedure is carried out by multiplying the stratum-specific antimicrobial use rate of the reference population by the number of patients in the corresponding stratum of each study hospital to generate an expected number of DOTs for each stratum. Expected DOTs are summed up across all strata to obtain the total expected number of DOTs for each hospital. The observed (O) antibiotic use is then compared with expected (E) use to arrive at the O/E ratio (See **Fig. 2**). A confidence interval is usually constructed around the O/E ratio and hospitals with a confidence interval that does not include unity are classified as outliers (see reference 32 for example).

---

adjusted expected use, as well as the observed to expected drug use in 35 clinical service lines (**Fig. 2**). We also found good agreement between direct and indirect standardization in ranking hospitals by their adjusted antibacterial drug use (weighted $\kappa = 0.85$, 95% confidence interval 0.78, 0.92).[43] Because this is a new method of risk adjustment applied to antimicrobial use, additional investigations should include both procedures to assess similarity in results.

AREAS IN WHICH MORE WORK IS NEEDED

Platt's comments about benchmarking health care–associated infections are also relevant to antimicrobial use: "We have made great progress since the CDC's landmark demonstrations of the utility of SSI surveillance to identify ways that hospitals can reduce their infection rates. It is important to do the new research needed to move surveillance from a research tool to one that can be widely used to support improved care."[36] The following are some of the research questions to be addressed so benchmarking will be useful to support improved patient care.

- Do hospital ASPs want to receive benchmarking data? When risk adjusted benchmarking reports (see **Fig. 2**) and summary statistics for antimicrobial drug use were offered to ASPs at 70 academic medical center hospitals among those in **Fig. 1**, only 50% of the hospitals responded (R.E. Polk, unpublished

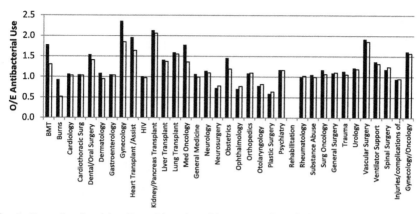

Fig. 2. Example of a risk adjusted benchmarking report for a hospital that compares the observed adult antibacterial drug use (O) with the expected (E) use in 35 clinical service lines. The solid bars are O/E ratios for DOT; the open bars are O/E ratios for LOT. Risk adjustment involved grouping each patient into 1 of the 35 clinical service lines based on their Medicare Severity Diagnosis Related Group (MS-DRG). Expected use was calculated by indirect standardization from antibacterial drug use during 2009 in 70 academic medical center hospitals (included in the 98 hospitals in **Fig. 1**). An O/E ratio greater than 1.0 suggests excessive use. The report also identified the reason(s) for excessive use, including excessive LOT/discharge compared with the benchmark, excessive use of combination therapies, or an excessive proportion of patients receiving antibacterial drugs. BMT, bone marrow transplant; HIV, human immunodeficiency virus. (*From* Polk RE, Hohmann SF, Medvedev S, et al. Benchmarking risk-adjusted adult antibacterial drug use in 70 US academic medical center hospitals. Clin Infect Dis 2011;53(11):1108; with permission.)

observations, 2012). If benchmarking is to become a useful tool, the information that is compelling to ASPs and most useful to support interventions must be identified.

- Do hospital ASPs act on receiving benchmarking data? Among the 50% of ASPs that requested benchmarking reports, it is unclear if any action resulted. For example, a hospital ASP that focuses on restriction and approval of specific high-dollar drugs may not be interested in a benchmarking report that focuses on excessive antimicrobial drug use in a clinical service area in which the financial impact may not be pronounced. It is also not clear what is the appropriate action step for a hospital that uses significantly fewer antibiotics than predicted. It is possible that patient outcomes or readmission rates from insufficiently treated infections are relatively unfavorable in these institutions; these outcomes should be explored in future work.
- Are hospital ASP interventions based on benchmarking data effective in changing antibiotic use? Do prescribing clinicians alter antimicrobial use when presented with benchmarking data? Do different clinical service areas (eg, orthopedics vs transplant services) respond differently to benchmarking data, perhaps influenced by perceived differences in patient SOI?
- Which kinds of interventions are most effective in improving antibiotic use? For example, when benchmarking suggests excessive antibiotic use in a clinical service, is the implementation of a clinical practice guideline more or less effective than concurrent review and feedback?

- If ASP interventions based on benchmarking reports are effective in changing antimicrobial use, does this result in improved clinical outcomes or reduced resistance? These most important outcomes are also the most difficult to determine.

THE OUTCOMES
Economic

Economic outcomes remain important to most programs and are the driving force supporting many programs. There have been many previous reviews of the economic benefits of stewardship; a common theme is that the cost savings of a new ASP are often dramatic in the first few years, but that savings plateau and may obscure a persistent economic benefit.[11,13,55] The economic impact after discontinuation of an established program was recently reported by Standiford and colleagues[13] from the University of Maryland. **Fig. 3** shows the economic benefit when starting the program, as well as the impact when the program was terminated. These data strongly suggest that this stewardship program was keeping a lid on expenses and show the dramatic effects when the lid was removed.

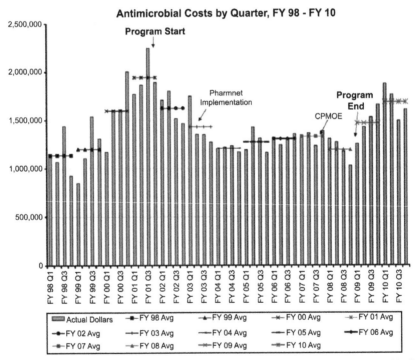

Fig. 3. Quarterly antimicrobial drug expenses at the University of Maryland hospital before initiation of the ASP (before Program Start *arrow*) and after implementation of the program until its termination (Program End *arrow*). The sudden increase in expenses after the program end is noteworthy. Vertical bars, quarterly costs; horizontal solid bars, fiscal year averages. CPMOE, computerized physician medication order entry; FY, financial year. (*From* Standiford HC, Chan S, Tripoli M, et al. Antimicrobial stewardship at a large tertiary care academic medical center: cost analysis before, during, and after a 7-year program. Infect Control Hosp Epidemiol 2012;33(4):340; with permission.)

Bacterial Resistance

Establishing cause and effect between a stewardship intervention and improved clinical outcomes, including rates of resistance, is challenging and may be more meaningful if evaluated at the patient level.[7,16] Different categories of resistance, such as multidrug resistance and extensive drug resistance, have been defined and standardized[56] and improvements in resistance have been linked to stewardship activities, particularly interventions to reduce antibiotic exposure and duration of therapy.[57] The design and interpretation of epidemiologic studies examining the association between antimicrobial use and resistance were recently reviewed by Schechner and colleagues[15]; **Box 3** summarizes the key methodologies.

Box 3
Methodological considerations for studies examining the association between antimicrobial use and resistance

Consideration for measuring resistance as an outcome of antimicrobial drug use

- The outcome can be defined as (1) presence or absence of resistance to a given antimicrobial agent (isolates with intermediate susceptibility may be considered resistant or susceptible), (2) change in minimum inhibitory concentration from its base value, or (3) mechanism by which resistance is conferred
- Whether the organism is resistant to 1 antimicrobial agent or multiple agents
- Type of specimens to be included (surveillance cultures, cultures collected during routine care, microbiologically and clinically documented infections, or site-specific cultures)
- The appropriate metric for measuring resistance; proportions are useful to clinicians, but rates are the recommended metric for measuring the burden of resistance and its association with antimicrobial use

Challenges in the design and analysis of the study

- Adjusting for confounding; this includes confounding by indication and the impact of infection control programs on antimicrobial resistance
- Establishing temporality between antimicrobial use and resistance

Choosing the appropriate study design

- Study designs that have been applied to analyze the impact of antimicrobial use on resistance include: (1) case control studies, (2) cohort studies, (3) ecological studies (4) quasiexperimental (pre-post) studies, (5) randomized controlled trials, and (6) studies based on mathematical modeling

Choosing the appropriate statistical method to adjust for confounding

- Methods commonly applied to control for confounding in studies on the association between antimicrobial use and resistance include: (1) multilevel (mixed model) analysis, (2) propensity scores, and (3) time series analysis

Adapted from Schechner V, Temkin E, Harbarth S, et al. Epidemiological interpretation of studies examining the effect of antibiotic usage on resistance. Clin Microbiol Rev 2013;26(2):289–307.

CDI

Others have summarized the positive impact on rates of CDI after ASP interventions in response to outbreaks of CDI.[58] What is less clear is the impact of routine ASP activities on the prevention of new CDI in the absence of an outbreak, and quantitative data regarding the interrelationship of ASP interventions and infection control efforts.

Suggestions that all new cases of CDI should be evaluated by the ASP to determine whether previous antimicrobial therapy was truly needed, and to devise corrective interventions (including education) if a systematic problem is found, seem to be reasonable ASP activities.[59–62] Furthermore, continuation of previous (non-CDI) antimicrobial therapy in the face of new onset CDI seems to be common,[59] and routine assessment of the need for continued antimicrobial treatment after CDI has been diagnosed should become an important ASP function. Benchmarking rates of CDI across multiple hospitals, identification of the causes of interhospital variability in rates, and the best strategies to reduce rates seem to be important areas for outcomes research.

SUMMARY

Measurement of inpatient antimicrobial use before and after ASP interventions and the associated outcomes should be core activities of a successful program. Measurement of antimicrobial drug use is becoming standardized and feasible in most institutions. To ensure the future of stewardship programs, outcomes from interventions must progress from economic measures to measures that document improved clinical outcomes, including lower rates of bacterial resistance. Benchmarking of antimicrobial use is recommended by most professional societies, but there are several questions that must be addressed before benchmarking is practical and a useful strategy to improve patient care. Despite some formidable challenges, the sophistication of stewardship program activities will likely increase as the science to support these programs continues to evolve.

ACKNOWLEDGMENTS

The authors wish to thank Drs Sam Hohmann and Saloni Kapur at the University HealthSystem Consortium (UHC) for their continued support by providing the data for **Fig. 1**. We also are grateful to the UHC hospital stewardship program personnel, who have been supportive of the research described in this review.

REFERENCES

1. Dellit TH, Owens RC, McGowan JE, et al. Infectious Diseases Society of America and the Society for Healthcare Epidemiology of America guidelines for developing an institutional program to enhance antimicrobial stewardship. Clin Infect Dis 2007;44(2):159–77.
2. Society for Healthcare Epidemiology of America, Infectious Diseases Society of America, Pediatric Infectious Diseases Society. Policy statement on antimicrobial stewardship by the Society for Healthcare Epidemiology of America (SHEA), the Infectious Diseases Society of America (IDSA), and the Pediatric Infectious Diseases Society (PIDS). Infect Control Hosp Epidemiol 2012;33(4):322–7.
3. Tamma PD, Cosgrove SE. Antimicrobial stewardship. Infect Dis Clin North Am 2011;25(1):245–60.
4. Drew RH, White R, MacDougall C, et al. Insights from the Society of Infectious Diseases Pharmacists on antimicrobial stewardship guidelines from the Infectious Diseases Society of America and the Society for Healthcare Epidemiology of America. Pharmacotherapy 2009;29(5):593–607.
5. Department of Health and Human Services, Office of Clinical Standards and Quality/Survey and Certification Group. Survey and certification focus on patient safety and quality–draft surveyor worksheets (October 14, 2011). Available at: http://. cdph.ca.gov////SurveyAndCertificationFocusDraftSurveyorWorksheetsCMSletter. pdf. Accessed November 11, 2013.

6. Morris AM, Brener S, Dresser L, et al. Use of a structured panel process to define quality metrics for antimicrobial stewardship programs. Infect Control Hosp Epidemiol 2012;33(5):500–6.
7. MacDougall C, Polk RE. Antimicrobial stewardship programs in health care systems. Clin Microbiol Rev 2005;18(4):638–56.
8. Griffith M, Postelnick M, Scheetz M. Antimicrobial stewardship programs: methods of operation and suggested outcomes. Expert Rev Anti Infect Ther 2012;10(1):63–73.
9. Jacob JT, Gaynes RP. Emerging trends in antibiotic use in US hospitals: quality, quantification and stewardship. Expert Rev Anti Infect Ther 2010;8(8): 893–902.
10. Ruef C. What's the best way to measure antibiotic use in hospitals? Infection 2006;34(2):53–4.
11. John JF, Fishman NO. Programmatic role of the infectious diseases physician in controlling antimicrobial costs in the hospital. Clin Infect Dis 1997;24(3): 471–85.
12. Goff DA, Bauer KA, Reed EE, et al. Is the "low-hanging fruit" worth picking for antimicrobial stewardship programs? Clin Infect Dis 2012;55(4):587–92.
13. Standiford HC, Chan S, Tripoli M, et al. Antimicrobial stewardship at a large tertiary care academic medical center: cost analysis before, during, and after a 7-year program. Infect Control Hosp Epidemiol 2012;33(4):338–45.
14. Johannsson B, Beekmann SE, Srinivasan A, et al. Improving antimicrobial stewardship: the evolution of programmatic strategies and barriers. Infect Control Hosp Epidemiol 2011;32(4):367–74.
15. Schechner V, Temkin E, Harbarth S, et al. Epidemiological interpretation of studies examining the effect of antibiotic usage on resistance. Clin Microbiol Rev 2013;26(2):289–307.
16. McGowan JE Jr. Antimicrobial stewardship—the state of the art in 2011: focus on outcome and methods. Infect Control Hosp Epidemiol 2012;33(4):331–7.
17. Centers for Disease Control and Prevention. Antibiotic resistance threats in the United States, 2013. Available at: http://.cdc.gov//report-2013/pdf/ar-threats-2013-508.pdf. Accessed November 11, 2013.
18. Boucher H, Talbot G, Bradley J, et al. Bad bugs, no drugs: no ESKAPE! An update from the Infectious Diseases Society of America. Clin Infect Dis 2009; 48(1):1.
19. Talbot GH, Bradley J, Edwards JE, et al. Bad bugs need drugs: an update on the development pipeline from the Antimicrobial Availability Task Force of the Infectious Diseases Society of America. Clin Infect Dis 2006;42(5):657–68.
20. Bad bugs, no drugs: as antibiotic discovery stagnates, a public health crisis brews. Arlington (VA): Infectious Diseases Society of America; 2004. Available at: http://.idsociety.org///policy_and_advocacy/_topics_and_issues/antimicrobial_resistance/10x20/images/bad_bugs_no_drugs.pdf. Accessed November 15, 2013.
21. The Donabedian model. Available at: http://En.wikipedia.org/wiki/_Donabedian_Model. Accessed November 11, 2013.
22. Solomkin JS, Mazuski JE, Bradley JS, et al. Diagnosis and management of complicated intra-abdominal infection in adults and children: guidelines by the Surgical Infection Society and the Infectious Diseases Society of America. Clin Infect Dis 2010;50(2):133–64.
23. Kullar R, Goff DA, Schulz LT, et al. The "Epic" challenge of optimizing antimicrobial stewardship: the role of electronic medical records and technology. Clin Infect Dis 2013;57(7):1005–13.

24. WHO Collaborating Centre for Drug Statistics Methodology. Guidelines for ATC classification and DDD assignment 2013. Oslo (Norway): 2012. Available at: http://.whocc.no///2013. Accessed November 15, 2013.

25. European Centre for Disease Prevention and Control. Surveillance of antimicrobial consumption in Europe, 2010. Stockholm (Sweden): ECDC; 2013. Available at: http://.ecdc.europa.eu////antibiotic-consumption-ESAC-report-2010-data.pdf. Accessed November 15, 2011.

26. Trivedi KK, Rosenberg J. The state of antimicrobial stewardship programs in California. Infect Control Hosp Epidemiol 2013;34(4):379–84.

27. Polk RE, Fox C, Mahoney A, et al. Measurement of adult antibacterial drug use in 130 US hospitals: comparison of defined daily dose and days of therapy. Clin Infect Dis 2007;44(5):664–70.

28. Schirmer PL, Mercier RC, Ryono RA, et al. Comparative assessment of antimicrobial usage measures in the Department of Veterans Affairs. Infect Control Hosp Epidemiol 2012;33(4):409–11.

29. Schwartz D, Evans RS, Camins B, et al. Deriving measures of intensive care unit antimicrobial use from computerized pharmacy data: methods, validation, and overcoming barriers. Infect Control Hosp Epidemiol 2011;32(5): 472–80.

30. Centers for Disease Control and Prevention. Antimicrobial use and resistance (AUR) module. Available at: http://www.cdc.gov/nhsn//pscManual/pscAURcurrent.pdf. Accessed November 11, 2013.

31. Fridkin SK, Srinivasan A. Implementing a strategy for monitoring inpatient antimicrobial use among hospitals in the United States. Clin Infect Dis 2014;58(3): 401–6.

32. Polk RE, Hohmann SF, Medvedev S, et al. Benchmarking risk-adjusted adult antibacterial drug use in 70 US academic medical center hospitals. Clin Infect Dis 2011;53(11):1100–10.

33. de With K, Maier L, Steib-Bauert M, et al. Trends in antibiotic use at a university hospital: defined or prescribed daily doses? Patient days or admissions as denominator? Infection 2006;34(2):91–4.

34. Filius PM, Liem TB, van der Linden PD, et al. An additional measure for quantifying antibiotic use in hospitals. J Antimicrob Chemother 2005;55(5):805–8.

35. Kuster SP, Ruef C, Ledergerber B, et al. Quantitative antibiotic use in hospitals: comparison of measurements, literature review, and recommendations for a standard of reporting. Infection 2008;36(6):549–59.

36. Platt R. Toward better benchmarking. Infect Control Hosp Epidemiol 2005;26(5): 433–4.

37. Ibrahim OM, Polk RE. Benchmarking antimicrobial drug use in hospitals. Expert Rev Anti Infect Ther 2012;10(4):445–57.

38. Rajmokan M, Morton A, Marquess J, et al. Development of a risk-adjustment model for antimicrobial utilization data in 21 public hospitals in Queensland, Australia (2006–11). J Antimicrob Chemother 2013;68(10):2400–5.

39. Amadeo B, Dumartin C, Robinson P, et al. Easily available adjustment criteria for the comparison of antibiotic consumption in a hospital setting: experience in France. Clin Microbiol Infect 2010;16(6):735–41.

40. MacDougall C, Polk RE. Variability in rates of use of antibacterials among 130 US hospitals and risk-adjustment models for interhospital comparison. Infect Control Hosp Epidemiol 2008;29(3):203–11.

41. Kuster SP, Ruef C, Bollinger AK, et al. Correlation between case mix index and antibiotic use in hospitals. J Antimicrob Chemother 2008;62(4):837–42.

42. Kanerva M, Ollgren J, Lyytikäinen O. Benchmarking antibiotic use in Finnish acute care hospitals using patient case-mix adjustment. J Antimicrob Chemother 2011;66(11):2651–4.
43. Ibrahim OM. Development and comparison of risk-adjusted models to benchmark antibiotic use in the University HealthSystem Consortium hospitals. 2012. Available at: https://.library.vcu.edu//handle/10156/4010/_Omar_PHD.pdf. Accessed November 11, 2013.
44. Norberg S, Struwe J, Grunewald M, et al. A pilot study of risk adjustment for benchmarking antibiotic use between hospitals in Sweden. J Glob Antimicrob Resist 2013. Available at: http://dx.doi.org/10.1016/j.jgar.2013.08.002. Accessed November 11, 2013.
45. Younger MS. Handbook for linear regression. North Scituate (MA): Duxbury Press; 1979.
46. Whittingham MJ, Stephens PA, Bradbury RB, et al. Why do we still use stepwise modelling in ecology and behaviour? J Anim Ecol 2006;75(5):1182–9.
47. Derksen S, Keselman HJ. Backward, forward and stepwise automated subset selection algorithms: frequency of obtaining authentic and noise variables. Br J Math Stat Psychol 1992;45(2):265–82.
48. Efron B, Hastie T, Johnstone I, et al. Least angle regression. Ann Stat 2004; 32(2):407–99.
49. Tibshirani R. Regression shrinkage and selection via the lasso. J R Stat Soc Series B Stat Methodol 1996;58(1):267–88.
50. Holland PW, Welsch RE. Robust regression using iteratively reweighted least-squares. Commun Stat Theory Methods 1977;6(9):813–27.
51. Shahian DM, Edwards FH, Jacobs JP, et al. Public reporting of cardiac surgery performance: part 2–implementation. Ann Thorac Surg 2011;92(3):S12–23.
52. Bailit J, Garrett J. Comparison of risk-adjustment methodologies for cesarean delivery rates. Obstet Gynecol 2003;102(1):45–51.
53. Narong MN, Thongpiyapoom S, Thaikul N, et al. Surgical site infections in patients undergoing major operations in a university hospital: using standardized infection ratio as a benchmarking tool. Am J Infect Control 2003;31(5): 274–9.
54. Shahian DM, Normand ST. Comparison of "risk-adjusted" hospital outcomes. Circulation 2008;117(15):1955–63.
55. Sick AC, Lehmann CU, Tamma PD, et al. Sustained savings from a longitudinal cost analysis of an internet-based preapproval antimicrobial stewardship program. Infect Control Hosp Epidemiol 2013;34(6):573–89.
56. Magiorakos AP, Srinivasan A, Carey RB, et al. Multidrug-resistant, extensively drug-resistant and pandrug-resistant bacteria: an international expert proposal for interim standard definitions for acquired resistance. Clin Microbiol Infect 2012;18(3):268–81.
57. Tamma PD, Turnbull AE, Milstone AM, et al. Ventilator-associated tracheitis in children: does antibiotic duration matter? Clin Infect Dis 2011;52(11):1324.
58. Feazel LM, Malhotra A, Perencevich EN, et al. Effect of antibiotic stewardship programmes on Clostridium difficile incidence: a systematic review and meta-analysis. J Antimicrob Chemother 2014. [Epub ahead of print].
59. Harpe SE, Inocencio TJ, Pakyz A, et al. Characterization of continued antibacterial therapy after diagnosis with nosocomial *Clostridium difficile* infection. Pharmacotherapy 2012;32(8):744–54.
60. Srigley JA, Brooks A, Sung M, et al. Inappropriate use of antibiotics and *Clostridium difficile* infection. Am J Infect Control 2013;41(11):1116–8.

61. Graber CJ, Madaras-Kelly K, Jones MM, et al. Unnecessary antimicrobial use in the context of *Clostridium difficile* infection: a call to arms for the Veterans Affairs Antimicrobial Stewardship Task Force. Infect Control Hosp Epidemiol 2013; 34(6):651–3.

62. Shaughnessy MK, Amundson WH, Kuskowski MA, et al. Unnecessary antimicrobial use in patients with current or recent *Clostridium difficile* infection. Infect Control Hosp Epidemiol 2013;34(2):109–16.

The Role of the Microbiology Laboratory in Antimicrobial Stewardship Programs

Edina Avdic, PharmD, MBA[a],*, Karen C. Carroll, MD[b]

KEYWORDS

- Antimicrobial stewardship • Microbiology laboratory • Rapid diagnostics
- Antibiogram • Procalcitonin

KEY POINTS

- Rapid diagnostic technologies can decrease the time to identification of microrganisms and resistance genes, potentially leading to reduced time to optimal therapy and improved clinical outcomes. The benefits of rapid diagnostic techniques are enhanced when coupled with antimicrobial stewardship interventions.
- Procalcitonin-guided therapy can reduce antimicrobial consumption by decreasing the initiation of antimicrobial therapy and decreasing the duration of therapy.
- Clinical microbiology laboratories should work closely with antimicrobial stewardship programs to compile institution-specific antibiograms. Antibiograms are frequently used by stewardship programs to make formulary decisions, develop guidelines for empiric therapy, and monitor local resistance rates over time.

INTRODUCTION

The major goals of antimicrobial stewardship programs (ASPs) are to optimize antimicrobial dosing, duration, and route of administration for each patient while minimizing adverse drug events and the emergence of antimicrobial resistance.[1,2] The clinical microbiology laboratory plays an essential role in these stewardship activities. Microbiology laboratories perform timely identification of microbial pathogens and antimicrobial susceptibility testing, and ensure proper attention to the preanalytical components of testing, which are often unrecognized tasks that can impact quality results. For example, most laboratories provide guidelines for appropriate specimen

Disclosures: Dr E. Avdic does not have disclosures. Dr K.C. Carroll has received research funding from BioFire Diagnostics, Inc, Nanosphere, Inc, and Curetis, Inc. She is on the scientific advisory boards of Quidel Biosciences, Inc and NanoMR, Inc.
[a] Department of Pharmacy, The Johns Hopkins Hospital, Osler 425, 600 North Wolfe Street, Baltimore, MD 21287, USA; [b] Departments of Pathology and Medicine, The Johns Hopkins University School of Medicine, Meyer B1-193, 600 North Wolfe Street, Baltimore, MD 21287, USA
* Corresponding author.
E-mail address: eavdic1@jhmi.edu

Infect Dis Clin N Am 28 (2014) 215–235
http://dx.doi.org/10.1016/j.idc.2014.01.002
0891-5520/14/$ – see front matter © 2014 Elsevier Inc. All rights reserved.

id.theclinics.com

collection, enforce rejection criteria for specimens inappropriately submitted, and have established procedures for limiting the work-up of contaminants (eg, blood cultures), all of which could impact antimicrobial use.[3] The preanalytical component of testing is not discussed in detail in this article and additional information can be found in the comprehensive document published by Baron and colleagues.[3]

The last decade has seen an unprecedented plethora of rapid, broad-based, and sensitive diagnostic tests that provide simultaneous organism identification and resistance marker detection. Optimal use of such assays provides tools that increase the effectiveness of antimicrobial stewardship (AS) activities and promote program growth.[4,5] Simultaneously laboratorians and ASP have pursued incorporating biomarkers, such as procalcitonin (PTC), into algorithms to differentiate infectious causes of fever or sepsis from noninfectious inflammatory conditions. Finally, clinical microbiology laboratories are essential for the surveillance of antimicrobial-resistant organisms and for organizing and communicating resistance trends in written form, such as antibiograms.

This article focuses primarily on the rapid tests that have been shown to optimize stewardship activities and reviews the evidence for using PTC. In addition, the value and limitations of antibiograms are also discussed in some detail.

RAPID DIAGNOSTIC TESTS FOR ORGANISM IDENTIFICATION

The past two decades have seen an explosion in the development of rapid diagnostic methods including nonamplified probe technologies, proteomics, and nucleic acid amplification methods combined with microarray technologies. A brief overview of several assays can be found in **Table 1**. These tests can significantly reduce time to organism identification compared with standard methods and lead to faster susceptibility results by detecting resistance markers. Moreover, when incorporated with AS interventions they can reduce the time to effective antimicrobial therapy, overall antimicrobial use, lengths of hospital stay, and hospital costs.[5–17] Summary of the studies evaluating rapid diagnostics can be found in **Table 2**.

Peptide Nucleic Acid–Fluorescence In Situ Hybridization

Peptide nucleic acid–fluorescence in situ hybridization (PNA-FISH) technology (AdvanDx, Inc, Woburn, MA) uses fluorescein-labeled probes that target pathogen-specific 16SrRNA of bacteria or 26SrRNA of yeast. After a blood culture bottle signals growth and a Gram stain is performed, the appropriate PNA-FISH probe can rapidly (20 minutes–1.5 hours) identify several important pathogens.[5] PNA-FISH probes have been cleared by the US Food and Drug Administration (FDA) for the following pathogens: *Staphylococcus aureus* and Coagulase-negative staphylococci; *Enterococcus faecalis* and other *Enterococcus* spp; *Escherichia coli*, *Klebsiella pneumonia*, and *Pseudomonas aeruginosa*; *Candida albicans*, *C parapsilosis*, *C tropicalis*, *C glabrata*, and *C krusei*. At this time, PNA-FISH tests do not detect resistance markers. However, a probe that detects the *mecA* gene has been evaluated in a recent clinical trial for FDA approval and will likely be available sometime in 2014 (Karen Carroll, personal communication, 2013).

Forrest and colleagues[6] conducted one of the first studies to evaluate the impact of a PNA FISH assay on patient outcomes. The investigators used an *S aureus* single-probe on positive blood cultures from non–intensive care unit (ICU) patients in conjunction with AS interventions. PNA-FISH results were reported in real time to an ASP that then assessed the need for vancomycin therapy and restricted its release. Investigators reported a significant decrease in median length of hospital stay from

Table 1
Features of select rapid diagnostic assays currently used in clinical practice

Technology	Manufacturer	Specimen	Organisms	Resistance Markers	Time Required (h)	FDA Cleared
PNA FISH	AdvanDx, Inc, Woburn, MA	Blood	Staphylococcus aureus/coagulase-negative staphylococci, Enterococcus faecalis/other Enterococcus spp, Escherichia coli/Klebsiella pneumoniae/Pseudomonas aeruginosa, Candida albicans/C parapsilosis/C tropicalis/C glabrata/C krusei	mecA[a]	0.3–1.5	Yes[a]
qPCR	BD GeneOhm, Inc, Sparks, MD; Cepheid, Sunnyvale, CA; Roche Molecular Systems, Inc, Indianapolis, IN	Blood, wounds	S aureus	mecA/SCCmec	1–2	Yes
MALDI-TOF MS	Bruker Daltonics, Inc, Billerica, MA; bioMerieux, Inc, Durham, NC	All body sites	Large number of organisms including bacteria and yeast	None	0.2	No
Nucleic acid microarray BC-GP	Nanosphere, Inc, Northbrook, IL	Blood	Staphylococcus spp, S aureus, S epidermidis, S lugdunensis; Streptococcus spp, S pneumoniae, S pyogenes, S agalactiae, S anginosus group; E faecalis, E faecium, Listeria spp	mecA, vanA, vanB	2.5	Yes
Nucleic acid microarray BC-GN	Nanosphere, Inc, Northbrook, IL	Blood	Escherichia coli/Shigella spp, Klebsiella pneumonia, Klebsiella oxytoca, P aeruginosa, Serratia marcescens, Acinetobacter spp, Proteus spp, Citrobacter spp, Enterobacter spp	KPC, NDM, CTX-M, VIM, IMP, OXA	2.5	Yes
Multiplex nucleic acid amplification test	BioFire, Inc, Salt Lake City, UT	Blood	Enterococcus spp, Listeria monocytogenes, Staphylococcus spp, S aureus, Streptococcus spp, S agalactiae, S pyogenes, S pneumoniae, A baumannii, Haemophilus influenzae, Neisseria meningitides, P aeruginosa, E cloacae complex, E coli, K oxytoca, K pneumoniae, S marcescens, Proteus spp, Enterobacteriaceae spp, C albicans, C parapsilosis, C tropicalis, C glabrata, C krusei	mecA, vanA, vanB, KPC	1	Yes

[a] Probe for mecA gene has been evaluated in a recent clinical trial, but not yet FDA approved.

Table 2
Studies evaluating rapid diagnostic tests for organism identification

Technology	Reference	Study Design	Organisms/ Antimicrobial Resistance Targets	AS-I	Impact on the Antimicrobial Therapy	Other Outcomes	Notes
PNA-FISH	Forrest et al,[6] 2006	Retrospective, cost-effective analysis comparing PNA-FISH result combined with AS interventions to historical control in patients with CoNS bacteremia	Staphylococcus aureus single probe	Yes	Nonsignificant trend toward less vancomycin use in non-ICU setting (4.9 DDD vs 6.78 DDD), and only 5% decrease in vancomycin use in ICU setting	Significant reduction in median length of stay (4 vs 6; $P<.05$) Decreased hospital costs, ~ $4000 per patient	
	Forrest et al,[7] 2006	Before and after design evaluating potential cost-savings of PNA-FISH result combined with AS in patients with candidemia	Single probe Candida albicans	Yes	Significant decrease in DDD/patient usage of caspofungin	Decrease in antifungal costs of $1729 per patient	Small sample
	Forrest et al,[8] 2008	Quasiexperimental study, pre and post PNA-FISH implementation with AS interventions in patients with GPCPC bacteremia	Enterococcus faecalis/ other Enterococcus spp	Yes	E faecalis: No difference in time to EAT (0.3 vs 0 d; $P = 1$) E faecium: Significantly shorter in PNA-FISH group (1.3 vs 3.1; $P<.001$)	LOS: no difference Decreased 30-day mortality in PNA-FISH group for patients with E faecum (26% vs 45%; $P = .04$), and no difference for E faecalis	

Study	Design	Probe/Organism	AS Combined	Antimicrobial Outcome	Clinical Outcome	Limitations
Ly et al,[18] 2008	Prospective, randomized controlled study comparing clinician notification of PNA-FISH results in patients with GPCC in blood	S aureus single probe	No	Antimicrobial use was reduced by 2.5 d (P = .01) in patients with CoNS, no difference in patients with S aureus	LOS: no difference. Median charges: $72,932 in PNA-FISH group vs $92,374 in usual care (P = .09). Overall reduced mortality PNA-FISH group (8 vs 17%; P = .05), but no difference when CoNS or S aureus were analyzed individually	Patients in usual care had higher comorbidity index compared to PNA FISH which may be confounder in patient outcomes
Holtzman et al,[19] 2011	Retrospective preintervention and postintervention study in patients with CoNS bacteremia	S aureus single probe	No	No significant difference in duration of vancomycin treatment (3.51 vs 4.15 d; P = .49)	Mean LOS: 20.9 vs 18.7 d; P = .35	
Heil et al,[11] 2012	Before and after design comparing PNA-FISH result combined with AS interventions to historical control in patients with candidemia	C albicans/C parapsilosis, C tropicalis, C glabrata/C krusei	Yes	Mean time to TT was significantly shorter in PNA-FISH group (0.6 vs 2.3 d; P = .0016)	Median time to culture clearance was significantly shorter (4 vs 5 d; P = .01) LOS: median 12 vs 25 (P = .82) No significant difference hospital mortality	Small sample size

(continued on next page)

Table 2
(continued)

Technology	Reference	Study Design	Organisms/ Antimicrobial Resistance Targets	AS-I	Impact on the Antimicrobial Therapy	Other Outcomes	Notes
qPCR	Carver et al,[9] 2008	Prospective two phase study Phase I results reported only Phase II results with AS intervention	*S aureus/mecA* and SCCmec from blood	Yes	Time to OAT decreased by 25.4 h		Sample was too small to evaluate other clinical outcomes
	Nguyen et al,[22] 2010	Retrospective comparative study, comparing qPCR with historical control in patients with MSSA and receiving vancomycin	*S aureus/mecA* and SCCmec from blood	No	Decrease in vancomycin usage from 3 to 1 d (*P*<.0001) Switch from vancomycin to β-lactam increased significantly (38.5%–61.7%; *P* = .004)	Hospitalization days decreased by median of 3 d (5 vs 8 d; *P* = .03)	

Bauer et al,[10] 2010	Nonequivalent study comparing pre-qPCR and post-qPCR with AS intervention	S aureus/mecA and SCCmec from blood	Yes	Shorter time to switch (1.7 d) from vancomycin to nafcillin/cefazolin for MSSA group (P = .02), no difference in MRSA group	Nonsignificant decrease in mean LOS by 6.2 d (P = .07) Mean hospital costs were decreased by $21,387 in rPCR group	qPCR was not independently associated with hospital mortality
Parta et al,[23] 2010	Retrospective comparative study, comparing qPCR with historical control	S aureus/mecA and SCCmec from blood	No	Significant decrease in the use of antistaphylococcal antibiotics for Staphylococcus spp other than S aureus (24% vs 45%; P<.01) Significantly shorter mean time OAT for MSSA (5.2 h vs 49.8 h; P = .007) Time to initiation of therapy for MRSA did not differ		

(continued on next page)

Table 2
(continued)

Technology	Reference	Study Design	Organisms/Antimicrobial Resistance Targets	AS-I	Impact on the Antimicrobial Therapy	Other Outcomes	Notes
MALDI-TOF MS	Huang et al,[14] 2013	Pre and post quasiexperimental study combined with real-time AS interventions	Gram-positive, gram-negative, yeast from blood	Yes	Time to EAT improved by 10 h in intervention group (20.4 h vs 30.1 h; $P = .021$) Time to OAT improved by 43 h in intervention group (47.3 h vs 90.3 h; $P<.001$)	Decreased ICU stay in intervention group (14.9 vs 8.3 d; $P = .014$) LOS: no difference (14.2 vs 11.4 d; $P = .66$) Mortality: 14.5% intervention vs 20.3% control ($P = .021$)	In multivariate regression analysis acceptance of AS intervention was not associated with reduced mortality
	Perez et al,[15] 2013	Preintervention and postintervention study coupled with real-time AS interventions	Gram-negatives from blood	Yes	At 24 h after bacteremia onset fewer patients were on inactive therapy in intervention cohort (4.7% vs 19.6%); Average time to initiation of active therapy was shorter in intervention cohort (36.5 h vs 73.2 h; $P<.001$)	LOS: significantly lower in the intervention cohort (9.3 vs 11.9; $P = .01$) Mean hospital costs were significantly lower in the intervention group ($26,162 vs $45,709; $P = .009$) Mortality: no difference (5.6% vs 10.7%)	Active therapy at 48 h and intervention were independently associated with decreased hospitalization

	Reference	Study design	Specimen		Results	Comments
	Vlek et al,[25] 2012	Preintervention and postintervention study	All positive blood cultures	No	11.3% increase in % of patients receiving appropriate antibiotic therapy 24 h after blood cultures turned positive (75.3% vs 64%; $P = .01$)	Other clinical outcomes were not evaluated
	Clerc et al,[13] 2013	Prospective observational study; all patients received infectious disease consultation	Gram-negatives from blood	No	Modifications in empiric therapy occurred in 35.1% patients; most frequent was early broadening of therapy (43.7%)	No comparative group; impact of antibiotic changes on clinical outcomes was not evaluated
qPCR + MALDI-TOF MS	Clerc et al,[17] 2013	Prospective, randomized open study comparing MALDI-TOF MS with MALDI-TOF MS + qPCR (results were reported to clinicians in both groups)	S aureus/mecA and SCCmec from blood	No	Nonsignificant decrease unnecessary glycopeptides coverage for MSSA (17.1% vs 29.2%; $P = .09$), when patients with PCN allergy were exclude decrease was significant (8.1% vs 26.1%; $P<.01$)	

(continued on next page)

Table 2
(continued)

Technology	Reference	Study Design	Organisms/ Antimicrobial Resistance Targets	AS-I	Impact on the Antimicrobial Therapy	Other Outcomes	Notes
Nucleic acid microarray (Verigene BC-GP)	Sango et al,[28] 2013	Pre and post quasiexperimental study	*Enterococcus* spp; *vanA, vanB*	Yes	Nonsignificant decrease in time to AAT for VSE (40.2 h vs 18.6; *P* = .115); Significant decrease in time to AAT for VRE (62.7 h vs 31.6 h; *P*<.0001)	LOS: significantly shorter 21.5 vs 43.2 d (*P* = .048). Not observed when deceased patients were removed I-LOS: no difference Costs: decrease in hospital costs by $60, 729 (*P* = .02) Infection related readmission w/90 d: no difference Attributed mortality: no difference	Patient groups were not matched

Abbreviations: AAT, appropriate antimicrobial therapy; AS-I, antimicrobial stewardship interventions; CoNS, coagulase-negative *staphylococci*; DDD, defined daily dose; EAT, effective antibiotic therapy; GPCC, gram-positive cocci in clusters; GPCPC, gram-positive cocci in pairs and chains; I-LOS, infection-related LOS; LOS, length of hospital stay; MRSA, methicillin-resistant *Staphylococcus aureus*; MSSA, methicillin-susceptible *S aureus*; OAT, optimal antibiotic therapy; TT, targeted therapy; VRE, vancomycin-resistant *Enterococcus*; VSE, vancomycin-sensitive *Enterococcus*.

6 to 4 days, a 5% reduction in vancomycin use, and overall hospital cost-savings of $4000 per patient. In a prospective randomized controlled study, Ly and colleagues[18] evaluated the impact of the PNA FISH S aureus/coagulase-negative staphylococci dual-probe on patient outcomes. The use of a laboratory clinical liaison that relayed the PNA FISH results to clinicians led to a reduction in mortality, from 16.8% to 7.9%, with the greatest impact on ICU patients. Antimicrobial use was reduced by an average of 2 days. A similar study demonstrated no observed benefit when the results were reported without active notification to clinicians.[19]

A 2-year quasiexperimental study demonstrated a significant reduction in time to effective therapy (1.3 vs 3.1 days) and 30-day mortality (26% vs 45%) in patients with *Enterococcus faecium* bacteremia using PNA-FISH technology with AS interventions.[8]

The role of PNA-FISH in the rapid identification of a variety of *Candida* spp from blood has demonstrated significant cost savings, mainly because of decrease in the use of expensive antifungal agents, such as echinocandins.[7,11,20] The use of PNA-FISH probes supplemented with clinician notification led to a cost savings of $1729 per patient.[7] Similarly, a potential cost savings of $1837 per patient was hypothesized by Alexander and colleagues[20] in a similar study. Heil and colleagues[11] found that when the results of a *Candida* PNA-FISH probe were combined with AS interventions that included calling the clinician with antifungal selection, dosage, and duration recommendations, there were significant decreases in time to targeted therapy (from 2.3 to 0.6 days), time to microbial clearance (from 5 to 4 days), and cost savings of $415 per patient. However, they were unable to demonstrate a difference in duration of hospital stay or mortality.[11]

Clinical outcomes studies using PNA-FISH probes distinguishing *P aeruginosa* from *E coli* and *K pneumoniae* have not yet been published.

Real-time Polymerase Chain Reaction Assays

Several quantitative polymerase chain reaction (qPCR) assays are available that can distinguish *S aureus* from other *Staphylococcus* spp and can identify the presence of methicillin-resistant genes (*mecA*, *SCCmec*) within 2 hours after cultures demonstrate microbial growth. These have largely been used for confirmation of positive blood cultures that contain gram-positive cocci in clusters and for rapid diagnosis of methicillin-resistant *S aureus* in wounds. The sensitivity of these assays approaches 100%.[5] Several commercial assays are available including the BD GeneOhm Staph SR (BD GeneOhm, Sparks, MD), Xpert MRSA/SA (Cepheid, Sunnyvale, CA), and the Light Cycler SeptiFast Test MGRADE (Roche Molecular Systems, Inc, Indianapolis, IN).[5,21] In some cases, clinical laboratories have developed their own assays.

In one study using a PCR test for *mecA* detection with active reporting of results for 46 patients with *S aureus* bacteremia, a 25-hour reduction in the time to optimal antimicrobial therapy was observed.[9] Nguyen and colleagues[22] showed that a laboratory-developed qPCR assay for methicillin-susceptible *S aureus* bacteremia led to a 2-day average decrease in days of vancomycin therapy and a 3-day decrease in length of hospital stay, even in the absence of concomitant AS interventions. Finally, in the study by Bauer and colleagues[10] incorporation of the Xpert MRSA/SA test, supplemented with AS interventions, decreased hospital costs by approximately $21,000.

Matrix-assisted Laser Desorption Ionization Time-of-flight Mass Spectrometry

Initially developed in 1980, matrix-assisted laser desorption ionization time-of-flight mass spectrometry (MALDI-TOF MS) has been routinely used throughout Europe for microbial identification and is now realizing widespread implementation in the

United States with recent FDA approval of the Bruker Biotyper (Bruker Daltonics, Inc, Billerica, MA) and the bioMerieux MS (bioMerieux, Inc, Durham, NC). Both systems provide rapid (0.2 hours) identification of a large number of organisms including bacteria and yeast recovered from cultures of different body sites.[12,24] Over the last 2 years several studies have evaluated the clinical impact of rapid organism identification by MALDI-TOF MS with or without AS interventions.

Huang and colleagues[14] conducted a quasiexperimental study to evaluate the impact of MALDI-TOF MS combined with real-time AS interventions in patients with bloodstream infections. They demonstrated decreases in time to organism identification, time to effective therapy, length of ICU stay, 30-day mortality, and recurrent bacteremia compared with a historic control group. Perez and colleagues[15] showed that MALDI-TOF MS in conjunction with AS interventions reduces the length of hospital stay (average of 2.6 days) and costs (average of $19,547) but were unable to show a reduction in mortality. Other investigators have similarly shown benefits with the use of MALDI-TOF.[13,16,17,25]

Broad-based Multiplexed Nucleic Acid Assays for Blood Culture Pathogen Identification

The Verigene blood culture gram-positive (BC-GP) nucleic acid test (Nanosphere, Inc, Northbrook, IL) uses a gold nanoparticle microarray to identify pathogenic gram-positive organisms, such as *Staphylococcus* spp, *S aureus*, *S epidermidis*, and *S lugdunensis*; *Streptococcus* spp, *S pneumoniae*, *S pyogenes*, *S agalactiae*, and *S anginosus* group; *E faecalis* and *E faecium*; and *Listeria* spp in positive blood cultures. The Verigene BC-GP test also detects the *mecA* (inferring methicillin resistance) and *vanA* and *vanB* (inferring vancomycin resistance). Use of this assay is limited to blood cultures and results are available approximately 2.5 hours after Gram stain identification.[26] Thus far this test has shown a high level of agreement when compared with conventional methods in its ability to quickly identify the previously mentioned pathogens and resistance markers.[26,27]

Sango and colleagues[28] evaluated the impact of the nucleic acid microarray assay combined with AS interventions on enterococcal bacteremia and showed a decrease in time to effective therapy, length of hospital stay (average of 21.7 days), and hospital costs ($60,729) compared with conventional methods. It is unclear whether similar benefits would be observed if used for all gram-positive organisms, which is more consistent with actual clinical practice. Nanosphere just received FDA clearance on an assay that identifies the following gram-negative organisms: *E coli* and *Shigella* spp; *K pneumonia*; *Klebsiella oxytoca*; *P aeruginosa*; *Serratia marcescens*; *Acinetobacter* spp; *Proteus* spp; *Citrobacter* spp; *Enterobacter* spp; and the resistance markers KPC, NDM, CTX-M, VIM, IMP, and OXA.

In addition to the Verigene BC-GP test, BioFire, Inc (Salt Lake City, UT) has a multiplex nucleic acid amplification test called the FilmArray BCID assay that identifies three genera and four species of gram-positive cocci, *Listeria monocytogenes*, *Proteus* spp, nine gram-negative rods to species level, and five species of yeasts.[29] In addition, it detects the following resistance determinants: *mecA*, *vanA*, *vanB*, and KPC. To date there are no publications on the impact of the FilmArray on AS interventions.

Before implementing any new rapid diagnostic test into a clinical microbiology laboratory, it is essential to pilot the test to determine any barriers to its use in the laboratory work flow and in clinician understanding and acceptance of the results. Additionally, a cost-effectiveness analysis that includes labor costs should be conducted. An ASP can be invaluable in rolling out new diagnostic tests by providing guidance on antimicrobial therapy and ensuring that therapy modifications are implemented in a timely manner. Any new laboratory test introduced into a clinical environment needs to be supplemented with education to clinicians to ensure that test results are interpreted appropriately. Results need to be reported in terms understandable to clinicians. Additionally, clinical support needs to be available to provide guidance and reassurance to providers.

PROCALCITONIN

PTC is a precursor peptide from the hormone calcitonin and a cytokine mediator that becomes elevated in bacterial infections and rapidly decreases during clinical recovery. PTC levels are virtually unchanged in viral infections.[30–32] In normal healthy subjects PTC has a plasma level of less than 0.1 μg/L and its elimination half-life ranges between 20 and 24 hours.[21,31] In the two meta-analyses PTC demonstrated superior diagnostic accuracy in severe infections compared with C-reactive protein.[33,34] A limitation of PTC is its elevation in response to a wide range of inflammatory conditions including pancreatitis, traumatic injury, major surgery, burns, and massive stress. Its production does not seem to be significantly mitigated by anti-inflammatory drugs.[31] Additionally, PTC can remain low in early or localized infection.[31,35] PTC is fairly expensive, with costs ranging from $30 to $47 per test.[36]

Use of PTC as a surrogate biomarker to guide antibiotic therapy has emerged in recent years. Previous prospective randomized trials evaluating PTC-guided therapy used algorithms with PTC cutoff ranges that guide clinicians when to initiate or discontinue therapy compared with control arms without PTC measurements.[37–51] Antimicrobial therapy is generally strongly discouraged for PTC levels less than 0.25 μg/L, discouraged for PTC less than 0.5 μg/L, encouraged for PTC greater than 0.5 μg/L, and strongly encouraged for PTC greater than or equal to 1 μg/L in most studies. If therapy is withheld PTC levels should generally be repeated 6 to 24 hours later, and if therapy is initiated they are repeated several times through the course of therapy, usually every 2 to 3 days to decide when to discontinue antibiotics. When PTC levels are very high at the beginning of therapy, discontinuation of therapy is usually encouraged when levels decline by 80% to 90% of the initial value. Because algorithm nonadherence has been shown to be a limitation in previous studies, routine reminders of the role of PTC should be emphasized.

Several randomized controlled trials have demonstrated that use of PTC can successfully reduce antimicrobial initiation and duration of therapy in acute respiratory tract infections in a variety of settings including primary care clinics, emergency departments, and hospital wards without negative impact on clinical outcomes.[37–44] Reduction in the duration of antimicrobial therapy has also been demonstrated in ICU patients with sepsis using PTC-guided therapy.[45–49]

PTC-guided Therapy in Acute Respiratory Tract Infections

PTC-guided therapy has been shown to reduce antibiotic prescriptions for upper respiratory tract infections by 42% and 72% in two multicenter randomized controlled trials conducted in the primary care setting, without compromising clinical outcomes.[40,42] PTC-guided therapy has similarly been shown to reduce antibiotic use in chronic obstructive pulmonary disease[39,44] and community-acquired pneumonia.[38,43,44]

A meta-analysis evaluating PTC use across all inpatient and outpatient settings found that PTC guidance was not associated with a decreased 30-day mortality compared with standard care (5.7% vs 6.3%) but did find that PTC-treated patients were at lower risk for treatment failure compared with control subjects (19.1% vs 21.9%; adjusted odds ratio, 0.82).[52]

PTC-guided Therapy in Critically Ill ICU Patients

Nobre and colleagues[45] used serial PTC measurement to determine the need for continued antibiotic therapy in patients with severe sepsis. They showed that PCT-guided therapy resulted in a 4-day reduction in the duration of antibiotic therapy (P = .003) and a 2-day reduction in ICU stay compared with the control group.[45] Similar findings were observed in several other smaller randomized trials in ICU patients with sepsis and ventilator-associated pneumonia, where a reduction in duration of antibiotic therapy ranged from 1.7 to 3.5 days with the use of PTC-guided therapy, without a negative impact on patient outcomes.[46–49]

However, two large, randomized controlled trials demonstrated no difference in antibiotic consumption when PTC-guided therapy algorithms were used[50,51] and suggest that these PTC may not be sensitive enough to distinguish infection from other noninfectious inflammatory conditions common in ICU patients including pancreatitis, trauma, and major surgery. A meta-analysis conducted by Wacker and colleagues[53] suggests that PTC has a sensitivity and specificity to diagnose bacterial sepsis in the range of 70% to 80% when a cutoff of 1 ug/L is used. At this time, because there are differing results in the use of PTC in critically ill patients, PTC should complement but not replace antimicrobial decision making in critically ill patients.

Although data are limited, the use of PTC seems promising in reducing the duration of antibiotic therapy in the neonatal and pediatric populations.[54,55] PTC has not been well studied in immunosuppressed patients and non–respiratory tract infections outside of ICU because those patients were generally excluded from studies. Existing studies have not incorporated AS interventions into evaluating the use of PTC-guided therapy. Although not formally evaluated, we believe ASPs can improve the use of PTC by developing diagnostic and treatment algorithms outlining how to incorporate PTC into clinical practice, particularly for outpatient and emergency department patients presenting with respiratory illnesses.

DEVELOPMENT OF ANTIBIOGRAMS

Antibiograms summarize the proportion of organisms that are susceptible to specific antimicrobials during a specified period of time, usually annually.[56] Antibiograms have several purposes. They provide guidance for clinicians with the selection of empiric antimicrobial therapy, they can be used to monitor antimicrobial resistance trends over time, and they provide useful information for formulary decisions.[1,56,57] Understanding the particulars of antibiograms is very important for ASPs and clinicians because they can obscure the actual local resistance rates and inaccurately reflect local antibiotic use.

The Clinical and Laboratory Standards Institute (CLSI) has developed consensus guidelines for the collection, analysis, and presentation of cumulative antibiograms in the United States (**Box 1**).[58] Adherence to the CLSI guidelines allows a more accurate assessment of intrainstitutional susceptibility patterns and interinstitutional benchmarking of susceptibility proportions.[59,60] In a recent survey of 49 academic medical centers and their affiliates, compliance with four key CLSI recommendations ranged from 64% to 98%.[61] In 16 hospitals (33%) formulary changes were made as a consequence of antibiogram results.[61] In a study including 55 hospitals generating pediatric antibiograms, most adhered to CLSI recommendations to update antibiograms at least annually (91%), eliminate duplicate cultures (91%), and exclude surveillance

---

Box 1
The Clinical and Laboratory Standards Institute recommendations for antibiogram development

Data should be stratified by:

 Patient population (inpatients, outpatients)

 Location (ICU, wards)

 Specimen types (all, blood, urine)

Data should include:

 Only species with at least 30 isolates

 Diagnostic isolates only (not surveillance)

 First isolate per patient in the period analyzed

 Results only for drugs that are routinely tested

Antibiograms should be generated at least annually

Data from Hindler JF, Stelling J. Analysis and presentation of cumulative antibiograms: a new consensus guideline from the Clinical and Laboratory Standards Institute. Clin Infect Dis 2007;44:867–73.

---

cultures (91%). The minority of institutions, however, required at least 30 isolates for each organism-antibiotic combination (16%); reported the preparation of unit-based antibiograms (38%); or reported separate antibiograms for urine isolates (38%), outpatients (27%), or patients with cystic fibrosis (31%). Only 16% of centers complied with all six CLSI recommendations for generation of antibiograms.[62]

Antibiogram Stratification by Location

Most institutions prepare institution-wide antibiograms for select clinically relevant pathogens and formulary antibiotics for a defined period of time. However, unit-specific data can be valuable in guiding empiric therapy choices. Binkley and colleagues[63] investigated differences between the susceptibility patterns reported in unit-specific and hospital-wide antibiograms over a 3-year period at their institution.[63,64] The investigators found that the percentages of antimicrobial-resistant organisms were significantly higher in the medical and surgical ICUs. When ICU data were included in the hospital-wide antibiogram, susceptibility patterns seemed significantly worse than when ICU data were reported separately.[63] These results are consistent with a previous study that found notable reductions in antimicrobial susceptibility proportions when ICU results were not reported separately.[64]

Similar to ICUs, a cumulative inpatient antibiogram may overestimate the degree of antimicrobial resistance found in the ambulatory setting, which can lead to prescribing of excessively broad-spectrum agents for community-acquired infections.[65,66] As a result, some institutions generate outpatient-specific antibiograms.

Combination Antibiograms

As the prevalence of resistance to some commonly prescribed antibiotics increases, particularly among gram-negative pathogens in critically ill patients, empiric combination therapy has become very important in clinical practice. As a result, the likelihood of selecting adequate empiric coverage by using combined antibiograms has been evaluated by several investigators.[67–69] Christoff and colleagues[67] have found that when a second agent was added to one of the backbone antipseudomonal agents for the treatment of five common gram-negative organisms in critically ill patients, there was a significant increase in the likelihood of covering the causative pathogen ($P<.01$). Similarly, Pogue and colleagues[68] found that combination antibiograms were able to predict optimal empiric combination regimens against all isolated gram-negative pathogens during a 6-month period in ICU patients with pneumonia.

Syndrome-specific Antibiograms

Syndrome-specific antibiograms have emerged in recent years because of the limited use of cumulative antibiograms in specific syndromes, such as intra-abdominal infections where multiple organisms are anticipated.[70,71] Hebert and colleagues[70] have created syndromic combination antibiograms at a four-hospital health system for abdominal-biliary and urinary tract infections. They further stratified syndrome-specific antibiograms based on patient characteristics (eg, nursing home residents) and have found considerable variability in adequacy of the empiric regimen depending on the patient risk factors. For example, ciprofloxacin would adequately cover urinary tract infections 82% of the time in otherwise healthy patients and only 20% in patients with fluoroquinolone exposure in the past 30 days.[70]

Use of Antibiograms in Constructing Empiric Regimen in Patients with Prolonged Hospital Stays

Unfortunately, most antibiograms used by hospitals do not take into consideration the timing of the infection, because according to CLSI guidelines, they include first clinical isolates of patients and do not reflect antimicrobial resistance that occurs during a hospitalization. Additionally, antibiograms fail to capture multidrug-resistant organisms because they provide percentage of susceptible isolates for individual antibiotics rather than all the antibiotics to which a particular organism was resistant.

Anderson and colleagues[72] conducted a retrospective cohort study to evaluate at what point during patients' hospital stays antibiograms no longer predict P aeruginosa susceptibility to commonly used antibiotics. The investigators found that standard antibiograms are unreliable for patients developing infections even within a week of hospitalization. The time to unreliability varied between ICU and non-ICU; it was significantly shorter in ICU patients.[72]

SUMMARY

Rapid diagnostic tests have been shown to lead to reductions in time to optimal antimicrobial therapy and improved patient outcomes, but their performance is greatly enhanced when an ASP is available to assist with education and real-time notification and interpretation of results. The periodic review of novel diagnostic tests should be conducted by the microbiology laboratory in conjunction with the ASP.

PTC-guided therapy can significantly reduce antibiotic consumption in acute respiratory tract infections without compromising patient outcomes. PTC-guided therapy also seems to have a beneficial role in reducing the duration of antimicrobial therapy for ICU patients with sepsis, but should complement and not replace other methods for determining antibiotic duration.

Antibiograms can assist ASPs with formulary decisions, guiding empiric therapy practices, and as a crude estimate for local resistance trends. Microbiology laboratories should generate at a minimum institutional, and if possible unit-specific antibiograms in accordance with CLSI guidelines. Microbiology laboratories are essential to ASPs by ensuring quality specimen collection, appropriate testing, implementation of rapid diagnostics, antimicrobial susceptibility testing, and data analysis.

REFERENCES

1. Dellit TH, Owens RC, McGowan JE, et al. Infectious Diseases Society of America and the Society for Healthcare Epidemiology of America guidelines for developing an institutional programs to enhance antimicrobial stewardship. Clin Infect Dis 2007;44:159–77.
2. Policy statement on antimicrobial stewardship by SHEA/IDSA/PIDS. Infect Control Hosp Epidemiol 2012;33:322–7.
3. Baron EJ, Miller JM, Weinstein MP, et al. Executive summary: a guide to utilization of the microbiology laboratory for diagnosis of infectious diseases: 2013 recommendations by the Infectious Diseases Society of America (IDSA) and the American Society of Microbiology (ASM). Clin Infect Dis 2013;57:485–8.
4. Bartlett JG, Gilbert DN, Spellberg G. Seven ways to preserve the miracle of antibiotics. Clin Infect Dis 2013;56:1445–50.
5. Goff DA, Jankowski C, Tenover FC. Using rapid diagnostic tests to optimize antimicrobial selection in antimicrobial stewardship programs. Pharmacotherapy 2012;32:677–87.
6. Forrest GN, Mehta S, Weekes E, et al. Impact of rapid in situ hybridization testing on coagulase-negative staphylococci positive blood cultures. J Antimicrob Chemother 2006;58:154–8.
7. Forrest NG, Mankes M, Jabra-Rizk A, et al. Peptide nucleic acid fluorescence in situ hybridization-based identification of *Candida albicans* and its impact on mortality and antifungal therapy costs. J Clin Microbiol 2006;44:3381–3.
8. Forrest GN, Roghmann MC, Toombs LS, et al. Peptide nucleic acid fluorescent in situ hybridization for hospital-acquired enterococcal bacteremia: delivering earlier effective antimicrobial therapy. Antimicrob Agents Chemother 2008;52:3558–63.
9. Carver PL, Lin S, DePestel DD, et al. Impact of mecA gene testing and intervention by infectious disease clinical pharmacists on time to optimal antimicrobial therapy for *Staphylococcus aureus* bacteremia at a university hospital. J Clin Microbiol 2008;46:2381–3.
10. Bauer KA, West JE, Balada-Llasat JM, et al. An antimicrobial stewardship program's impact with rapid polymerase chain reaction methicillin-resistant *Staphylococcus aureus*/*S. aureus* blood culture test in patients with *S. aureus* bacteremia. Clin Infect Dis 2010;51:1076–80.
11. Heil EL, Daniels LM, Long DM, et al. Impact of a rapid peptide nucleic acid fluorescence in situ hybridization assay on treatment of *Candida* infections. Am J Health Syst Pharm 2012;69(21):1910–4.
12. Tan KE, Ellis BC, Lee R, et al. Prospective evaluation of a matrix-assisted laser desorption ionization-time of flight mass spectrometry system in a hospital clinical microbiology laboratory for identification of bacteria and yeasts: a bench-by-bench study for assessing the impact on time to identification and cost-effectiveness. J Clin Microbiol 2012;50:3301–8.
13. Clerc O, Prodhom G, Vogne C, et al. Impact of matrix-assisted laser desorption ionization time-of-flight mass spectrometry on the clinical management of patients with gram-negative bacteremia: a prospective observational study. Clin Infect Dis 2013;56:1101–7.
14. Huang AM, Newton D, Kunapuli A, et al. Impact of rapid organism identification via matrix-assisted laser desorption/ionization time-of-flight combined with antimicrobial stewardship team intervention in adult patients with bacteremia and candidemia. Clin Infect Dis 2013;57:1237–45.

15. Perez KK, Olsen RJ, Musick WL, et al. Integrating rapid pathogen identification and antimicrobial stewardship significantly decreases hospital costs. Arch Pathol Lab Med 2013;137(9):1247–54.

16. Tamma PD, Tan K, Nussenblatt VR, et al. Can matrix-assisted laser desorption ionization time-of-flight mass spectrometry (MALDI-TOF) enhance antimicrobial stewardship efforts in the acute care setting? Infect Control Hosp Epidemiol 2013;34(9):990–5.

17. Clerc O, Prod'hom G, Senn L, et al. Matrix-assisted laser desorption ionization time-of-flight mass spectrometry and PCR-based rapid diagnosis of Staphylococcus aureus bacteraemia. Clin Microbiol Infect 2013. [Epub ahead of print].

18. Ly T, Gulia J, Pyrgos V, et al. Impact upon clinical outcomes of transplant of PNA FISH-generated laboratory data from the clinical microbiology bench to bedside in real time. Ther Clin Risk Manag 2008;4:637–40.

19. Holtzman C, Whitney D, Barlam T, et al. Assessment of impact of peptide nucleic acid fluorescence in situ hybridization for rapid identification of coagulase-negative staphylococci in the absence of antimicrobial stewardship intervention. J Clin Microbiol 2011;49:1581–2.

20. Alexander BD, Ashley ED, Reller LB, et al. Cost savings with implementation of PNA FISH testing for identification of Candida albicans in blood cultures. Diagn Microbiol Infect Dis 2006;54(4):277–82.

21. Riedel S, Carroll KC. Laboratory detection of sepsis: biomarkers and molecular approaches. Clin Lab Med 2013;33:413–37.

22. Nguyen DT, Yeh E, Perry S, et al. Real-time PCR testing for mecA reduces vancomycin usage and length of hospitalization for patients infected with methicillin-sensitive staphylococci. J Clin Microbiol 2010;48(3):785–90.

23. Parta M, Goebel M, Thomas J, et al. Impact of an assay that enables rapid determination of Staphylococcus species and their drug susceptibility on the treatment of patients with positive blood culture results. Infect Control Hosp Epidemiol 2010;31(10):1043–8.

24. Patel R. Matrix-assisted laser desorption ionization-time of flight mass spectrometry in clinical microbiology. Clin Infect Dis 2013;57(4):564–72.

25. Vlek AL, Bonten MJ, Boel CH. Direct matrix-assisted laser desorption ionization time-of-flight mass spectrometry improves appropriateness of antibiotic treatment of bacteremia. PLoS One 2012;7:e32589.

26. Scott LJ. Verigene® gram-positive blood culture nucleic acid test. Mol Diagn Ther 2013;17(2):117–22.

27. Alby K, Daniels LM, Weber DJ, et al. Development of a treatment algorithm for streptococci and enterococci from positive blood cultures identified with the verigene gram-positive blood culture assay. J Clin Microbiol 2013;51(11):3869–71.

28. Sango A, McCarter YS, Johnson D, et al. Stewardship approach for optimizing antimicrobial therapy through use of a rapid microarray assay on blood cultures positive for Enterococcus species. J Clin Microbiol 2013;51(12):4008.

29. Blaschke AJ, Heyrend C, Byington CL, et al. Rapid identification of pathogens from positive blood cultures by multiplex polymerase chain reaction using the FilmArray system. Diagn Microbiol Infect Dis 2012;74:349–55.

30. Müller B, Becker KL, Schächinger H, et al. Calcitonin precursors are reliable markers of sepsis in a medical intensive care unit. Crit Care Med 2000;28(4):977–83.

31. Schuetz P, Christ-Crain M, Müller B. Procalcitonin and other biomarkers to improve assessment and antibiotic stewardship in infections: hope for hype? Swiss Med Wkly 2009;139(23–24):318–26.

32. Riedel S. Procalcitonin and the role of biomarkers in the diagnosis of sepsis. Diagn Microbiol Infect Dis 2012;73:221–7.
33. Simon L, Gauvin F, Amre DK, et al. Serum procalcitonin and C-reactive protein levels as markers of bacterial infection: a systematic review and meta-analysis. Clin Infect Dis 2004;39(2):206–17.
34. Uzzan B, Cohen R, Nicolas P, et al. Procalcitonin as a diagnostic test for sepsis in critically ill adults and after surgery or trauma: a systematic review and meta-analysis. Crit Care Med 2006;34(7):1996–2003.
35. Agarwal R, Schwartz DN. Procalcitonin to guide duration of antimicrobial therapy in intensive care units: a systematic review. Clin Infect Dis 2011;53(4): 379–87.
36. Smith KJ, Wateska A, Nowalk MP, et al. Cost-effectiveness of procalcitonin-guided antibiotic use in community acquired pneumonia. J Gen Intern Med 2013;28(9):1157–64.
37. Christ-Crain M, Jaccard-Stolz D, Bingisser R, et al. Effect of procalcitonin-guided treatment on antibiotic use and outcome in lower respiratory tract infections: cluster-randomised, single-blinded intervention trial. Lancet 2004; 363(9409):600–7.
38. Christ-Crain M, Stolz D, Bingisser R, et al. Procalcitonin guidance of antibiotic therapy in community-acquired pneumonia: a randomized trial. Am J Respir Crit Care Med 2006;174(1):84–93.
39. Stolz D, Christ-Crain M, Bingisser R, et al. Antibiotic treatment of exacerbations of COPD: a randomized, controlled trial comparing procalcitonin-guidance with standard therapy. Chest 2007;131(1):9–19.
40. Briel M, Schuetz P, Mueller B, et al. Procalcitonin-guided antibiotic use vs a standard approach for acute respiratory tract infections in primary care. Arch Intern Med 2008;168(18):2000–7.
41. Kristoffersen KB, Søgaard OS, Wejse C, et al. Antibiotic treatment interruption of suspected lower respiratory tract infections based on a single procalcitonin measurement at hospital admission: a randomized trial. Clin Microbiol Infect 2009;15(5):481–7.
42. Burkhardt O, Ewig S, Haagen U, et al. Procalcitonin guidance and reduction of antibiotic use in acute respiratory tract infection. Eur Respir J 2010;36(3):601–7.
43. Long W, Deng X, Zhang Y, et al. Procalcitonin guidance for reduction of antibiotic use in low-risk outpatients with community-acquired pneumonia. Respirology 2011;16(5):819–24.
44. Schuetz P, Christ-Crain M, Thomann R, et al. Effect of procalcitonin-based guidelines vs standard guidelines on antibiotic use in lower respiratory tract infections: the ProHOSP randomized controlled trial. JAMA 2009;302(10): 1059–66.
45. Nobre V, Harbarth S, Graf JD, et al. Use of procalcitonin to shorten antibiotic treatment duration in septic patients: a randomized trial. Am J Respir Crit Care Med 2008;177(5):498–505.
46. Stolz D, Smyrnios N, Eggimann P, et al. Procalcitonin for reduced antibiotic exposure in ventilator-associated pneumonia: a randomised study. Eur Respir J 2009;34(6):1364–75.
47. Hochreiter M, Köhler T, Schweiger AM, et al. Procalcitonin to guide duration of antibiotic therapy in intensive care patients: a randomized prospective controlled trial. Crit Care 2009;13(3):R83.
48. Schroeder S, Hochreiter M, Koehler T, et al. Procalcitonin (PCT)-guided algorithm reduces length of antibiotic treatment in surgical intensive care patients

with severe sepsis: results of a prospective randomized study. Langenbecks Arch Surg 2009;394(2):221–6.

49. Bouadma L, Luyt CE, Tubach F, et al. Use of procalcitonin to reduce patients' exposure to antibiotics in intensive care units (PRORATA trial): a multicentre randomised controlled trial. Lancet 2010;375(9713):463–74.

50. Layios N, Lambermont B, Canivet JL, et al. Procalcitonin usefulness for the initiation of antibiotic treatment in intensive care unit patients. Crit Care Med 2012; 40(8):2304–9.

51. Jensen JU, Hein L, Lundgren B, et al. Procalcitonin-guided interventions against infections to increase early appropriate antibiotics and improve survival in the intensive care unit: a randomized trial. Crit Care Med 2011;39(9):2048–58.

52. Schuetz P, Briel M, Christ-Crain M, et al. Procalcitonin to guide initiation and duration of antibiotic treatment in acute respiratory infections: an individual patient data meta-analysis. Clin Infect Dis 2012;55(5):651–62.

53. Wacker C, Prkno A, Brunkhorst FM, et al. Procalcitonin as a diagnostic marker for sepsis: a systematic review and meta-analysis. Lancet Infect Dis 2013; 13(5):426–35.

54. Baer G, Baumann P, Buettcher M, et al. Procalcitonin guidance to reduce antibiotic treatment of lower respiratory tract infection in children and adolescents (ProPAED): a randomized controlled trial. PLoS One 2013;8(8):e68419.

55. Stocker M, Fontana M, El Helou S, et al. Use of procalcitonin-guided decision-making to shorten antibiotic therapy in suspected neonatal early-onset sepsis: prospective randomized intervention trial. Neonatology 2010;97:165–74.

56. Leuthner KD, Doern GV. Antimicrobial stewardship programs. J Clin Microbiol 2013;51(12):3916–20.

57. Schulz LT, Fox BC, Polk RE. Can the antibiogram be used to assess microbiologic outcomes after antimicrobial stewardship interventions? A critical review of the literature. Pharmacotherapy 2012;32(8):668–76.

58. Hindler JF, Stelling J. Analysis and presentation of cumulative antibiograms: a new consensus guideline from the Clinical and Laboratory Standards Institute. Clin Infect Dis 2007;44:867–73.

59. Zapantis A, Lacy MK, Horvat RT, et al. Nationwide antibiogram analysis using NCCLS M39-A guidelines. J Clin Microbiol 2005;43(6):2629–34.

60. Boehme MS, Somsel PA, Downes FP. Systematic review of antibiograms: a National Laboratory System approach for improving antimicrobial susceptibility testing practices in Michigan. Public Health Rep 2010;125(Suppl 2):63–72.

61. Xu R, Polk RE, Stencel L, et al. Antibiogram compliance in University HealthSystem Consortium participating hospitals with Clinical and Laboratory Standards Institute guidelines. Am J Health Syst Pharm 2012;69:598–606.

62. Tamma PD, Robinson GL, Gerber JS, et al. Pediatric antimicrobial susceptibility trends across the United States. Infect Control Hosp Epidemiol 2013;34(12): 1244–51.

63. Binkley S, Fishman NO, LaRosa LA, et al. Comparison of unit-specific and hospital-wide antibiograms: potential implications for selection of empirical antimicrobial therapy. Infect Control Hosp Epidemiol 2006;27(7):682–7.

64. Kaufman D, Haas CE, Edinger R, et al. Antibiotic susceptibility in the surgical intensive care unit compared with the hospital-wide antibiogram. Arch Surg 1998;133:1041–5.

65. McGregor JC, Bearden DT, Townes JM, et al. Comparison of antibiograms developed for inpatients and primary care outpatients. Diagn Microbiol Infect Dis 2013;76(1):73–9.

66. Dahle KW, Korgenski EK, Hersh AL, et al. Clinical value of an ambulatory-based antibiogram for uropathogens in children. J Pediatric Infect Dis Soc 2012;1(4): 333–6.
67. Christoff J, Tolentino J, Mawdsley E, et al. Optimizing empirical antimicrobial therapy for infection due to gram-negative pathogens in the intensive care unit: utility of a combination antibiogram. Infect Control Hosp Epidemiol 2010; 31(3):256–61.
68. Pogue JM, Alaniz C, Carver PL, et al. Role of unit-specific combination antibio-grams for improving the selection of appropriate empiric therapy for gram-negative pneumonia. Infect Control Hosp Epidemiol 2011;32(3):289–92.
69. Fox BC, Shenk G, Peterson D, et al. Choosing more effective antimicrobial com-binations for empiric antimicrobial therapy of serious gram-negative rod infec-tions using a dual cross-table antibiogram. Am J Infect Control 2008;36:S57–61.
70. Hebert C, Ridgway J, Vekhter B, et al. Demonstration of the weighted-incidence syndromic combination antibiogram: an empiric prescribing decision aid. Infect Control Hosp Epidemiol 2012;33:381–8.
71. Davis ME, Anderson DJ, Sharpe M, et al. Constructing unit-specific empiric treatment guidelines for catheter-related and primary bacteremia by deter-mining the likelihood of inadequate therapy. Infect Control Hosp Epidemiol 2012;33(4):416–20.
72. Anderson DJ, Miller B, Marfatia R, et al. Ability of an antibiogram to predict Pseudomonas aeruginosa susceptibility to targeted antimicrobials based on hospital day of isolation. Infect Control Hosp Epidemiol 2012;33(6):589–93.

Antimicrobial Stewardship in Long-term Care Facilities

Susan M. Rhee, MD[a],*, Nimalie D. Stone, MD, MS[b]

KEYWORDS

- Long-term care • Antimicrobial stewardship • Antimicrobial resistance • Elderly
- Infection prevention

KEY POINTS

- Long-term care facilities (LTCF) house a unique patient population, who are often elderly with several preexisting medical conditions.
- Residents of LTCF are often colonized with multidrug-resistant organisms, and antibiotic stewardship is essential to limit the further emergence of resistance.
- Antimicrobial stewardship is a new but necessary concept in LTCFs.
- Stewardship strategies from acute care settings may be adapted to function with the available resources utilized in LTCFs.

INTRODUCTION

Antimicrobial resistance has been identified as a major public health crisis. National summary data from the Centers for Disease Control and Prevention (CDC) estimate that more than 2 million illnesses are attributable to resistant infections.[1] As a result of increasing prevalence of virulent and drug-resistant organisms, including *Clostridium difficile*, methicillin-resistant *Staphylococcus aureus* (MRSA), and drug-resistant gram-negative organisms, there has been a call for the implementation of antimicrobial stewardship programs (ASPs) across the health care spectrum.[2] ASP refers to the development of programs that addresses the "appropriate selection, dosing, route, and duration of antimicrobial therapy". Guidelines for the development of stewardship programs generally target stewardship activities in the acute care setting.[3] The success of stewardship programs in the hospital setting has been described, with reductions in the rate of *C. difficile* infection, antibiotic usage, and improved pharmacy expenditures.[4–6] Implementation of similar programs in

Disclosures: The findings and conclusions in this report are those of the authors and do not necessarily represent the official position of the Centers for Disease Control and Prevention.
[a] Division of Infectious Diseases, Johns Hopkins Bayview Medical Center, 5200 Eastern Avenue, MFL Center Tower, 3rd Floor, Baltimore, MD 21224, USA; [b] Division of Healthcare Quality Promotion, Centers for Disease Control and Prevention, 1600 Clifton Road Northeast, MS:A-31, Atlanta, GA 30333, USA
* Corresponding author.
E-mail address: srhee9@jhmi.edu

Infect Dis Clin N Am 28 (2014) 237–246
http://dx.doi.org/10.1016/j.idc.2014.01.001
0891-5520/14/$ – see front matter © 2014 Elsevier Inc. All rights reserved.

long-term care facilities (LTCF) has been limited, despite the heavy use of antibiotics and high prevalence of resistant organisms in these settings.[7] To add to an already complicated picture, the population in the United States continues to age, with an estimated 21% of the population in 2040 consisting of adults 65 years of age and older.[8] As increased usage of LTCFs looms, the burden of inappropriate usage of antimicrobials in this health care setting will also increase in the absence of appropriate guidance.

THE BURDEN OF INFECTION IN LTCF

There are more than 15,000 nursing homes in the United States, with an estimated 1.5 million residents.[9] Previous epidemiologic studies have reported an infection prevalence rate of 5.3%, based on a single-day survey, and infection incidence rates ranging from 3.6 to 5.2/1000 resident days.[10–12] The most commonly reported infections in nursing homes are urinary tract infections (UTIs), lower respiratory tract infections, including pneumonia, skin and soft tissue infections, and gastroenteritis. Infections are among the most frequent causes of transfer to acute care hospitals, and 30-day hospital readmissions from LTCF are associated with increased mortality in this population.[13–16]

The burden of multidrug-resistant organisms has also been identified as a key issue in this population, often a consequence of the overuse of antibiotics.[17] There is a higher incidence of invasive MRSA in adults greater than or equal to 65 years old, as compared with their younger counterparts.[18] Surveillance of various facilities has shown high prevalence of both colonization and infection with resistant organisms such as MRSA and multidrug-resistant gram-negative pathogens.[19–21] Among LTCF residents, infections with antibiotic-resistant organisms are associated with more severe infection, hospitalization, increased risk of death, and increased cost of care.[22–24] With a growing population of residents transferring between hospitals and LTCFs, the risk for resistance to emerge and spread within LTCFs has increased. In a study assessing movement of patients between health care settings, more than 50% of individuals identified with a carbapenem-resistant organism during a hospitalization were discharged to post-acute care facilities such as LTCFs.[25] Failure to control spread of resistance in LTCFs can also affect surrounding hospitals. An MRSA outbreak in one LTCF led to increasing prevalence of this organism in several adjacent California hospitals.[26]

The antimicrobial overuse in LTCF exposes residents to the potential and realized harm that is caused by antibiotics, such as C. difficile infection.[27–29] In a study of nursing homes in Rhode Island, 72% of patients received an antibiotic that was inappropriate according to established guidelines, with 67% receiving antibiotic therapy longer than the recommended duration, with a resultant increased incidence of C. difficile infection. In the geriatric population, it has already been shown that antimicrobials are one of the most commonly prescribed medications, with a significant associated adverse drug event risk.[29]

CHALLENGES WITH ANTIMICROBIAL USE IN LTCF

ASPs in LTCFs have to address the unique challenges in identifying and managing infections in this population. The prevalence of asymptomatic bacteriuria (ASB) ranges from 23% to 50% in noncatheterized LTCF residents, to 100% among those with long-term urinary catheters, and ASB in the older adult is accompanied by pyuria in more than 90% of cases.[30] However, symptomatic UTIs in LTCF residents may present atypically. A study assessing the clinical signs and symptoms of older adults (older than 75 years) with bacteremic UTIs found that 10/37 (27%) did not mount a fever greater than 37.9°C, and 48.6% failed to report any localizing urinary tract symptoms (eg, dysuria, urgency, or frequency).[31] Given the unreliable clinical assessment for infections in LTCF residents and the diagnostic challenges in differentiating ASB from infection, suspected UTIs account for 30% to 60% of antibiotic prescriptions in LTCFs.[32,33]

Adding to the challenge of diagnosing infections in LTCF is having clinical providers located off-site, and making management decisions based on the assessments communicated by front-line staff. The use of surrogate assessments and the lack of access to provider follow-up likely drive antibiotic use and frequent hospital transfers. Many facilities have limited diagnostic testing (eg, laboratory or radiology) available, with services contracted to off-site facilities leading to delays in obtaining specimens, processing, and reporting results back to providers.

PATTERNS OF ANTIMICROBIAL USE IN LTCF

Antimicrobials, specifically antibiotics, are among the most frequently prescribed medications in LTCFs and have the second highest rate of adverse drug events following antipsychotic medications.[34,35] In a study of antimicrobial use in 73 nursing homes, the pooled mean rate was 4.8 antimicrobial courses/1000 resident days (range 0.4–23.5).[32] Other studies have shown that 47% to 79% of LTCF residents are exposed to at least one antibiotic course over a 12-month period.[7,36] Factors accounting for the facility-level variability in antimicrobial use may include provider prescribing habits, types of resident services provided within the facility (eg, custodial LTCF vs post-acute skilled), and resident case-mix index.[37–39] Estimates on the amount of inappropriate antimicrobial use in LTCFs vary widely, from 25% to 75%, depending on how appropriateness is defined.[34,40]

To guide health care practitioners in the rational assessment of infections in this vulnerable population, clinical guidelines have been published, which outline the evaluation for residents suspected of having an infection.[41] Minimum criteria that should be present before initiating antimicrobial therapy, known as the "Loeb criteria", have also been proposed to improve antimicrobial use (**Box 1**).[42] Surveillance definitions for infections in LTCFs, referred to as the "McGeer criteria", have also been published to support infection surveillance activities in LTCF (**Box 2**).[43,44] However, despite the creation of these guidance documents to assist clinicians with the diagnosis and management of common infections, the implementation of these guidelines remains a challenge. One study showed that only 12.7% of prescriptions were adherent to the Loeb criteria within 12 nursing home evaluations.[36] A cluster, randomized controlled trial, which operationalized diagnostic and therapeutic algorithms based on the Loeb criteria for the management of UTI in 24 nursing homes, found a 31% reduction in antimicrobial use for UTI among intervention homes compared with controls.[33] However, despite a reduction in antibiotic use for UTI, the overall antibiotic consumption did not differ between the 2 groups, suggesting that use may have shifted to other indications. Continued inappropriate treatment of infections that do not meet clinical criteria has been attributed to the perception of the need to treat, despite the lack of objective evidence.[45]

IMPLEMENTING ANTIMICROBIAL STEWARDSHIP INTERVENTIONS IN LTCFS

ASP refers to the development of programs that addresses the "appropriate selection, dosing, route, and duration of antimicrobial therapy".[3,46,47] Recently, CDC outlined core elements for hospital antibiotic stewardship program that can be tailored to the infrastructure and capacity of different sized facilities, including LTCFs. The core elements emphasized leadership commitment, accountability for improving antibiotic use, need for drug expertise, implementing action through targeted policies and

Box 1
Loeb minimum criteria for the initiation of antibiotics in long-term care facility residents

Skin and Soft Tissue Infections

New or increasing purulent drainage and/or ≥2 of the following:

Fever

Temperature >37.9°C (100°F) or

Increase of 1.5°C (2.4°F) from baseline temperature

Redness

Tenderness

Warmth

New or increasing swelling of the affected site

Respiratory infections

In residents with temperature >38.9°C (102°F), ≥1 of the following:

Respiratory rate >25 breaths/min

Productive cough

In residents with temperature >37.9°C (100°F), but ≤38.9°C (102°F)

Cough and ≥1 of the following:

Pulse >100 beats/min

Delirium

Rigors

Respiratory rate >25

In afebrile residents with chronic obstructive pulmonary disease and age >65 years old

New or increased cough with purulent sputum production

In afebrile residents without chronic obstructive pulmonary disease

New cough with purulent sputum production and ≥1 of the following:

Respiratory rate >25

Delirium

Urinary Tract Infections

Without indwelling urinary catheters

Acute dysuria or

Fever (>37.9°C [100°F]) and ≥1 of the following:

New or worsening urgency

Frequency

Suprapubic pain

Gross hematuria

Costovertebral angle tenderness

Urinary incontinence

With chronic indwelling urinary catheter

≥1 of the following

Fever (>37.9°C [100°F])

New costovertebral angle tenderness

Rigors

New onset delirium

Fever without obvious focus of infection

Fever (>37.9°C [100°F]) and ≥1 of the following

New onset of delirium

Rigors

Data from Loeb M, Bentley D, Bradley S, et al. Development of minimum criteria for the initiation of antibiotics in residents of long-term-care facilities: results of a consensus conference. Infect Control Hosp Epidemiol 2001;22:120–4.

Box 2
Definitions included in the McGeer and Revised McGeer criteria

Respiratory tract infections

Common cold syndromes/pharyngitis

Influenzalike illness

Pneumonia

Other lower respiratory tract infections

Urinary tract infections

Eye, ear, nose, and mouth infections

Conjunctivitis

Ear infection

Mouth/perioral infections

Sinusitis

Skin infections

Cellulitis/soft tissue/wound infections

Fungal skin infections

Herpes simplex, herpes zoster infections

Scabies

Gastrointestinal tract illnesses

Gastroenteritis

Norovirus

Clostridium difficile infection

Systemic infections

Primary bloodstream infections

Unexplained febrile episodes

Data from McGeer A, Campbell B, Emori TG, et al. Definitions of infection for surveillance in long-term care facilities. Am J Infect Cont 1991;19(1):1–7; and Stone ND, Ashraf M, Calder J, et al. Surveillance definitions of infections in longterm care facilities: revisiting the McGeer criteria. Infect Control Hosp Epidemiol 2012;33(10):965–77.

guidelines, tracking and reporting to staff on prescribing and resistance, and offering education.[48] Recommendations for infection prevention and control in the LTCF setting include using ASP as part of the ongoing infection prevention program.[40,49]

The staffing structure within LTCFs may be considerably different from acute care facilities, with the largest proportion of in-person staffing consisting of nursing, with variable models of physician presence. Although some facilities maintain their own internal physician staffing models, many have physicians who are off site and unable to interact with LTCF residents on a daily basis, leading to dependence on nursing staff, often nursing assistants, for the initial recognition of signs and symptoms suggestive of infection. As the request for diagnostic testing and antimicrobial prescriptions are often called in by the physician before having the opportunity to examine the patient, education about diagnostic criteria and appropriate culture techniques need to occur at all levels of staffing. Identifying key participants and ASP champions is essential to initiating change within an institution. At a minimum, consider engaging the following nursing home personnel in the implementation of any stewardship activities: administrative leadership, clinical leadership including the medical director and the director of nursing services, the infection prevention and control coordinator, the consultant pharmacist, as well as representatives from the medical and nursing staff. Although including an infectious disease (ID) specialist would be ideal, including any physician with an interest in antimicrobial stewardship may be a more practical approach, especially in areas where ID specialists are not readily available. Senior level nursing may be able to provide the front-line support in assuring adherence to guidelines for initial diagnostic procedures, whereas post-prescription review of antibiotic therapy may be performed by a physician or pharmacist if available.

Management Strategies

A baseline evaluation of the quantity of antimicrobials prescribed expressed as days of therapy per 1000 patient days, to allow for interfacility comparison, should be conducted. Further evaluation into the use of specific agents and their indications should occur to determine which stewardship interventions are most necessary.

Existing guidelines for antimicrobial use developed by IDSA and SHEA should be tailored to meet local needs. Any guideline needs to be supplemented with education to ensure proper dissemination and use. Materials and methods to initiate an antimicrobial stewardship program may include

- Sessions with the ASP team and the providers of care, to educate on a more personal basis, which may provide an avenue for prescribers to directly ask questions.
- Antibiotic dosing guidelines to be created based on a facility's formulary, which would be readily available to prescribers, with information on drug interactions as part of the guidelines, given the frequency of polypharmacy in this population.
- Educational modules for nursing assistants and nursing staff on the criteria for initiation of antimicrobial usage.
- Educational modules for residents and family members, given that there can be pressure applied to the prescriber to give an inappropriate antimicrobial, when one is not indicated, due to external pressure exerted.
- Diagnostic and treatment guidelines can be adapted from currently published sources on common infectious problems, such as pneumonia, UTIs, and skin and soft tissue infections, and made available to all pertinent care-giving staff.
- Guidelines and educational modules focusing on preventable problems that also lead to infection may also be a part of an LTCF stewardship program; for example, following best practices for infection control, prevention of pressure

ulcer formation, and aspiration prevention will avoid the infectious complications that often follow.

By engaging several different educational strategies, important and applicable guideline information can be disseminated in a fairly easy manner, although retention of the material requires repeated education campaigns.

PREPRESCRIPTION AUTHORIZATION

With preprescription authorization, physicians contact a stewardship team before prescribing select antimicrobials. Preprescription authorization ensures that patients receive the most appropriate empiric antimicrobial therapy and reduces the number of unnecessary antimicrobial starts. Unfortunately, it can be resource intensive in real time and may lead to delays in the initiation of therapy. This may be particularly true in LTCF where clinicians are often off site.

POST-PRESCRIPTION REVIEW WITH FEEDBACK

Post-prescription review with feedback entails a review of antimicrobials prescribed at some time point after more clinical and microbiology laboratory information is available. Although it usually occurs at 48 to 72 hours, it can occur at any time period and still proves valuable even if it occurs once or twice a week because of limited resources. As there is greater flexibility in the timing of interventions with post-prescription review and feedback, this may be more feasible in LTCFs. Feedback likely requires phone calls or secure e-mails to providers as notes left in charts are unlikely to be seen in a timely manner.

SUCCESSFUL ANTIMICROBIAL STEWARDSHIP INTERVENTIONS IN LTCFS

Although still relatively new in LTCF settings, the impact of such an ASP has already demonstrated positive results. The implementation of such programs led to a 30% decrease in systemic antibiotic usage, both in oral and intravenous medications, in addition to a decrease in the rate of positive *C. difficile* tests, in one institution.[50] Although this study used an ID service, simply distributing appropriate educational material targeting the most common infections in LTCFs has shown to improve antibiotic usage, as demonstrated by Monette and colleagues[51]; a 20% decrease in prescriptions that were not adherent to guidelines was seen in the group of prescribers who were given the educational material, as opposed to control.

Areas of Future Needed Work

- Robust studies examining the efficacy of various programs and how they fit into individual facility types with differing resources.
- Attention to the issues of transmission between the LTCFs and the acute care facilities serving the same community.
- Increased implementation of the nationally available guidelines in LTCFs.

SUMMARY

The selection pressure resulting from the overuse of antibiotics is a significant driver of adverse events in the LTCF setting. In addition, as patients move back and forth between acute care and long-term care, the burden of multidrug resistance and frequent infections is shared across the health care spectrum. By adapting stewardship principles that have already been shown to be effective in the acute care setting to LTCFs, an impact can be made on the health of the overall population and in this vulnerable population.

REFERENCES

1. Centers for Disease Control and Prevention. Antibiotic resistance threats in the United States, 2013. Atlanta (GA): Centers for Disease Control and Prevention; 2013. Available at: http://www.cdc.gov/drugresistance/threat-report-2013/pdf.
2. Bartlett JG. A call to arms: the imperative for antimicrobial stewardship. Clin Infect Dis 2011;53(1):S4–7.
3. Dellit TH, Owens RC, McGowan JE, et al. Infectious Diseases Society of America and the Society for Healthcare Epidemiology of America guidelines for developing an institutional program to enhance antimicrobial stewardship. Clin Infect Dis 2007;44:159–77.
4. Malani AN, Richards PG, Kapila S, et al. Clinical and economic outcomes from a community hospital's antimicrobial stewardship program. Am J Infect Control 2013;41(2):145–8.
5. Aldeyab MA, Kearney MP, Scott MG, et al. An evaluation of the impact of antibiotic stewardship on reducing the use of high-risk antibiotics and its effect on the incidence of Clostridium difficile infection in hospital settings. J Antimicrob Chemother 2012;67(12):2988–96.
6. Goff DA, Bauer KA, Reed EE, et al. Is the "low hanging fruit" worth picking for antimicrobial stewardship programs? Clin Infect Dis 2012;55(4):587–92.
7. Van Buul LW, van der Steen JT, Veenhuizen RB, et al. Antibiotic Use and Resistance in Long Term Care Facilities. J Am Med Dir Assoc 2012;13: 568.e1–13.
8. Administration on Aging. A profile of older Americans. Washington, DC: Department of Health & Human Services, Administration on Aging; 2012. Available at: http://www.aoa.gov/AoARoot/Aging_Statistics/Profile/2012/4.aspx. Accessed September, 2013.
9. FastStats. CDC. Available at: http://www.cdc.gov/nchs/fastats/nursingh.htm. Accessed September 1, 2013.
10. Tsan L, Langberg R, Davis C, et al. Nursing home-associate infection in Department of Veterans Affairs community living centers. Am J Infect Control 2010; 38(6):461–6.
11. Stevenson KB, Moore J, Colwell H, et al. Standardized infection surveillance in long-term care: interfacility comparisons from a regional cohort of facilities. Infect Control Hosp Epidemiol 2005;26:231–8.
12. Koch AM, Eriksen HM, Elstrøm P, et al. Severe consequences of healthcare-associated infections among residents of nursing homes: a cohort study. J Hosp Infect 2009;71:269–74.
13. Teresi JA, Holmes D, Bloom HG, et al. Factors differentiating hospital transfers from long-term care facilities with high and low transfer rates. Gerontologist 1991;31:795–806.
14. Ouslander JG, Diaz S, Hain D, et al. Frequency and diagnoses associated with 7- and 30-day readmission of skilled nursing facility patients to a nonteaching community hospital. J Am Med Dir Assoc 2011;12:195–203.
15. Boockvar KS, Gruber-Baldini AL, Burton L, et al. Outcomes of infection in nursing home residents with and without early hospital transfer. J Am Geriatr Soc 2005;53:590–6.

16. Ahmed AA, Hays CL, Liu B, et al. Predictors of in-hospital mortality among hospitalized nursing home residents: an analysis of the National Hospital Discharge Surveys 2005-2006. J Am Med Dir Assoc 2010;11:52–8.
17. Loeb MB, Craven S, McGeer A, et al. Risk factors for resistance to antimicrobial agents among nursing home residents. Am J Epidemiol 2003;157:40–7.
18. Centers for Disease Control and Prevention. Active Bacterial Core Surveillance Report, Emerging Infections Program Network, Methicillin-Resistant *Staphylococcus aureus*, 2011. Atlanta (GA): Centers for Disease Control and Prevention; 2011. Accessed September 2013.
19. Rogers MA, Mody L, Chenoweth C, et al. Incidence of antibiotic-resistant infection in long-term residents of skilled nursing facilities. Am J Infect Control 2008; 36:472–5.
20. O'Fallon E, Pop-Vicas A, D'agata E. The emerging threat of multidrug-resistant gram-negative organisms in long-term care facilities. J Gerontol A Biol Sci Med Sci 2009;64A(1):138–41.
21. Furano JP, Hebden J, Standiford H, et al. Prevalence of methicillin-resistant *Staphylococcus aureus* and *Acinetobacter baumanii* in a long-term acute care facility. Am J Infect Control 2008;36:468–71.
22. Ma HM, Wah JL, Woo J. Should nursing home-acquired pneumonia be treated as nosocomial pneumonia? J Am Med Dir Assoc 2012;13(8):727–31.
23. Suetens C, Niclaes L, Jans B, et al. Methicillin-resistant Staphylococcus aureus colonization is associated with higher mortality in nursing home residents with impaired cognitive status. J Am Geriatr Soc 2006;54(12):1854–60.
24. Capitano B, Nicolau DP. Evolving epidemiology and cost of resistance to antimicrobial agents in long-term care facilities. J Am Med Dir Assoc 2003;4:S90–9.
25. Perez F, Endimiani A, Ray AJ, et al. Carbapenem-resistant Acinetobacter baumannii and Klebsiella pneumonia across a hospital system: impact of post-acute care facilities on dissemination. J Antimicrob Chemother 2010;65:1807–18.
26. Lee BY, Bartsch SM, Wong KF, et al. The Importance of Nursing Homes in the Spread of Methicillin-resistant *Staphylococcus aureus* (MRSA) Among Hospitals. Med Care 2013;51:205–15.
27. Rotjananpan P, Dosa D, Thomas K. Potentially inappropriate treatment of urinary tract infections in two rhode island nursing homes. Arch Intern Med 2011;171(5): 438–43.
28. Juthani-Mehta M, Tinetti M, Perrelli E, et al. Diagnostic accuracy of criteria for urinary tract infection in a cohort of nursing home residents. J Am Geriatr Soc 2007;55:1072–7.
29. Gerwitz JH, Field TS, Harrold LR. Incidence and preventability of adverse drug events among older persons in the ambulatory settting. JAMA 2003;289: 1107–11.
30. Juthani-Mehta M. Asymptomatic bacteriuria and urinary tract infection in older adults. Clin Geriatr Med 2007;23:585–94.
31. Woodford HJ, Graham C, Meda M, et al. Bacteremic urinary tract infections in hospitalized older patients – are any currently available diagnostic criteria sensitive enough? J Am Geriatr Soc 2011;59:567–8.
32. Benoit SR, Nsa W, Richards CL, et al. Factors associated with antimicrobial use in nursing homes: a multilevel model. J Am Geriatr Soc 2008;56:2039–44.
33. Loeb M, Brazil K, Lohfield L, et al. Effect of a multifaceted intervention on number of antimicrobial prescriptions for suspected urinary tract infections in residents of nursing homes: cluster randomised controlled trial. British Med J 2005;331:669.

34. Nicolle LE, Bentley DW, Garibaldi R, et al. Antimicrobial use in long-term-care facilities. SHEA Long-Term-Care Committee. Infect Control Hosp Epidemiol 2000;21:537–45.

35. Gurwitz JH, Field TS, Avorn J, et al. Incidence and preventability of adverse drug events in nursing homes. Am J Med 2000;109:87–94.

36. Olsho LE, Bertrand RM, Edwards AS, et al. Does adherence to the loeb minimum criteria reduce antibiotic prescribing rates in nursing homes? J Am Med Dir Assoc 2013;14:309.e1–7.

37. Richards CL Jr, Darradji M, Weinberg A, et al. Antimicrobial use in post-acute care: a retrospective descriptive analysis in seven long-term care facilities in Georgia. J Am Med Dir Assoc 2005;6:109–12.

38. Mylotte JM, Keagle J. Benchmarks for antibiotic use and cost in long-term care. J Am Geriatr Soc 2005;53:1117–22.

39. Mylotte JM, Neff M. Trends in antibiotic use and cost and influence of case-mix and infection rate on antibiotic-prescribing in a long-term care facility. Am J Infect Control 2003;31:18–25.

40. Smith PW, Watkins K, Miller H, et al. Antibiotic stewardship programs in long-term care facilities. Ann Longterm Care 2011;19:20–5.

41. High KP, Bradley SF, Gravenstein S, et al. Clinical practice guideline for the evaluation of fever and infection in older adult residents of long-term care facilities: 2008 update by the Infectious Diseases Society of America. J Am Geriatr Soc 2009;57:375–94.

42. Loeb M, Bentley D, Bradley S, et al. Development of minimum criteria for the initiation of antibiotics in residents of long-term-care facilities: results of a consensus conference. Infect Control Hosp Epidemiol 2001;22:120–4.

43. McGeer A, Campbell B, Emori TG, et al. Definitions of infection for surveillance in long-term care facilities. Am J Infect Control 1991;19:1–7.

44. Stone ND, Ashraf M, Calder J, et al. Surveillance definitions of infections in long-term care facilities: revisiting the McGeer criteria. Infect Control Hosp Epidemiol 2012;33(10):965–77.

45. Walker S, McGeer A, Simor AE, et al. Why are antibiotics prescribed for asymptomatic bacteriuria in institutionalized elderly people? A qualitative study of physicians' and nurses' perceptions. Can Med Assoc J 2000;163:273–7.

46. Moody J, Cosgrove SE, Olmsted R, et al. Antimicrobial stewardship: a collaborative partnership between infection preventionists and health care epidemiologists. Am J Infect Control 2012;40(2):94–5.

47. MacDougal C, Polk RE. Antimicrobial stewardship programs in health care systems. Clin Microbiol Rev 2005;18(4):638–56.

48. CDC. Core Elements of Hospital Antibiotic Stewardship Programs. Atlanta (GA): US Department of Health and Human Services, CDC; 2014. Available at: http://www.cdc.gov/getsmart/healthcare/implementation/core-elements.html.

49. Smith PW, Bennett G, Bradley S, et al. SHEA/APIC Guideline: infection prevention and control in the long-term care facility. Am J Infect Control 2008;36:504–35.

50. Jump RL, Olds DM, Seifi N, et al. Effective antimicrobial stewardship in a long-term care facility through an infectious disease consultation service: keeping a LID on antibiotic use. Infect Control Hosp Epidemiol 2012;33(12):1185–92.

51. Monette J, Miller MA, Monette M, et al. Effect of an educational intervention on optimizing antibiotic prescribing in long-term care facilities. J Am Geriatr Soc 2007;55:1231–5.

Antimicrobial Stewardship in the NICU

Joseph B. Cantey, MD[a,b,*], Sameer J. Patel, MD, MPH[c]

KEYWORDS

- Neonatal intensive care unit • Stewardship • Antimicrobial • Metrics

KEY POINTS

- Neonatologists care for a population at high risk for sepsis who present with very nonspecific signs and symptoms.
- Neonates often receive prolonged antibiotic therapy for treatment of culture-negative sepsis.
- Multidisciplinary collaboration and meaningful antibiotic stewardship metrics for neonatologists are necessary.
- Key stewardship interventions include collection of appropriate blood cultures, use of ancillary laboratory tests, avoidance of unnecessarily broad empiric therapy, and de-escalation or discontinuation therapy.
- Future efforts should include coordinating with other quality-improvement efforts and building a stewardship research infrastructure.

INTRODUCTION: NATURE OF THE PROBLEM
Adverse Outcomes Related to Antibiotic Use

Antibiotics are the most commonly prescribed medications in neonatal intensive care units (NICUs).[1] There is increasing evidence that inappropriate or excessive use of antibiotics in the NICU leads to serious adverse outcomes. These outcomes include the emergence of multidrug-resistant organisms (MDROs), linked to endemic or epidemic infections[2–4]; increased rates of invasive candidiasis[5–7]; necrotizing enterocolitis (NEC); late-onset sepsis (LOS); or death (**Table 1**).[8–10]

[a] Division of Pediatric Infectious Disease, Department of Pediatrics, University of Texas Southwestern Medical Center, 5323 Harry Hines Boulevard, Dallas, TX 75390, USA; [b] Division of Neonatal/Perinatal Medicine, Department of Pediatrics, University of Texas Southwestern Medical Center, 5323 Harry Hines Boulevard, Dallas, TX 75390, USA; [c] Division of Pediatric Infectious Diseases, Department of Pediatrics, Ann & Robert H. Lurie Children's Hospital of Chicago Northwestern University Feinberg School of Medicine, 225 East Chicago Avenue, Box 20, Chicago, Illinois 60611–2605, USA
* Corresponding author. Division of Pediatric Infectious Disease, Department of Pediatrics, University of Texas Southwestern Medical Center, 5323 Harry Hines Boulevard, Dallas, TX 75390.
E-mail address: Joseph.Cantey@UTSouthwestern.edu

Infect Dis Clin N Am 28 (2014) 247–261
http://dx.doi.org/10.1016/j.idc.2014.01.005
0891-5520/14/$ – see front matter © 2014 Elsevier Inc. All rights reserved.

id.theclinics.com

Table 1
Adverse events associated with antibiotic use in the NICU

Study	Population	Antibiotic Exposure	Adverse Event	Odds Ratio (95% Confidence Interval)
Cotten et al,[8] 2007	5693 ELBW infants in 19 centers (NICHD NRN)	≥5 d of initial empiric therapy despite sterile cultures	NEC or death NEC Death	1.50 (1.22–1.83) 1.34 (1.04–1.73) 1.86 (1.45–2.39)
Kuppala et al,[9] 2011	365 VLBW infants, 3 centers	≥5 d of initial empiric therapy despite sterile cultures	NEC, LOS, or death LOS	2.66 (1.12–6.30) 2.45 (1.28–4.67)
Cotten et al,[5] 2006	3702 ELBW infants in 12 centers (NICHD NRN)	Any receipt of third-generation cephalosporin or carbapenem	Invasive candidiasis	Hazard ratio 1.68
Saiman et al,[7] 2001	370 ELBW infants in 6 centers	Any receipt of third-generation cephalosporin	Candida colonization	1.85 (1.24–2.77)
Lee et al,[6] 2013	530,162 infants >1500 g	Any receipt of third-generation cephalosporin, carbapenems, ticarcillin, or piperacillin	Invasive candidiasis	1.6 (1.10–2.40)
de Man et al,[4] 2000	436 infants in 2 centers	Crossover trial of cefotaxime vs tobramycin for empiric therapy	Colonization with organism resistant to empiric therapy	18.0 (5.6–58.0) for cefotaxime exposure

Abbreviations: ELBW, extremely low birth weight (<1000 g); NICHD NRN, National Institute for Child Health and Human Development Neonatal Research Network.

Alteration of the neonatal microbiome by antibiotic exposure has been suggested as a mechanism for some of these adverse effects.[11] Infants treated with antibiotics experience a decrease in genetic diversity of their microbiome and a surge in Proteobacteria along with a reduction in Firmicutes.[12,13] Mai and colleagues[11] demonstrated a similar bloom in Proteobacteria within 7 days of an episode of NEC in their case-control study of infants less than 32 weeks' gestation. Although it is unclear whether altering the concentration of Proteobacteria or Firmicutes plays a causal role, it is becoming clear that changes to the microbiome are associated with an increased risk for NEC. Furthermore, serial genetic analysis of the infant microbiome has shown that the acquisition of resistant bacteria begins at birth and can be driven by systemic antibiotic therapy.[14] These alterations to the infant microbiome can lead to poor outcomes not only for that infant but also other infants in the intensive care unit because of the horizontal transmission of pathogens.[15]

Diagnostic Challenges

The predominant challenge to antibiotic stewardship in the NICU is that sepsis in the neonate can present with nonspecific findings, and many of these findings overlap widely with noninfectious causes.[16] A normal physical examination does not exclude bacteremia,[17] and at present there is no combination of laboratory testing with sufficient sensitivity to preclude infection. As a result, there is a very low threshold for neonatologists to obtain cultures and start empiric therapy for clinical signs that could be consistent with sepsis. Clinical signs including apnea, respiratory distress, tachycardia, and temperature instability are not very specific in diagnosing sepsis.[18] Not surprisingly, uninfected infants with respiratory distress syndrome[19] or transient tachypnea of the newborn[20] are frequently treated with empiric antibiotic therapy pending their culture results. Hypotension is another finding that may lead to empiric antibiotic therapy. Up to 20% of infants who are less than 1500 g experience hypotension, a rate tenfold higher than their incidence of sepsis.[21]

Culture-Negative Sepsis

A diagnostic dilemma occurs when cultures are sterile but the infant continues to have clinical signs or abnormal laboratory values that could be consistent with sepsis. There are 2 common situations that lead to the treatment of culture-negative sepsis. First, many preterm infants have clinical signs that are caused by their prematurity but are indistinguishable from sepsis, such as respiratory distress and hypotension. These infants are more likely to receive prolonged antibiotic therapy despite sterile cultures. Second, when mothers receive intrapartum antibiotic prophylaxis (IAP), some providers think that such antibiotic therapy might mask a true sepsis episode by making the infant's blood culture falsely negative.[22] Maternal IAP is highly effective in preventing neonatal sepsis and is intended to ensure that infants have sterile cultures.[23] Therefore, these infants actually are at a lower, not higher, risk for sepsis because of maternal IAP.

The duration of therapy for culture-negative sepsis varies widely between and within centers, and studies have shown that the duration of therapy may not be related to the infant's clinical findings or risk factors for sepsis.[24] Cordero and Ayers[24] performed a study of 790 infants who were less than 1000 g who received empiric antibiotics for early onset sepsis (EOS) and had sterile blood cultures. The duration of antibiotic therapy did not correlate with the number of risk factors for EOS or Clinical Risk Index in Babies (CRIB-I) scores, a validated severity score for preterm infants.[25] Spitzer and colleagues[26] reported a cohort of 998 term neonates treated for suspected EOS who, by 24 hours of age, were on full feeds and had normal vital signs and sterile blood cultures. Infants with no risk factors received a median of 3.3 days of antibiotics; infants with 2 or more risk factors received a median of 3.5 days. Despite sterile cultures and no clinical signs of sepsis, greater than 20% of infants in the cohort received 5 or more days of therapy.

Variation in Treatment Duration for Infections

Treatment variation in the NICU persists even if infection is diagnosed. In a study from Liem and colleagues[27] describing a survey of antibiotic use in the Netherlands, 10 units had 7 different empiric regimens for LOS, 6 for meningitis, and 7 for NEC. Antibiotic use in the highest-volume NICU was almost 3 times higher than the use in the lowest-volume NICU despite similar patient populations. It is clear that centers manage clinical scenarios in a variety of ways. For pneumonia, this problem is exacerbated by the challenge of differentiating pneumonia from other causes of respiratory distress in the newborn in a timely manner. Protocols that use objective risk factors in combination with culture results and clinical course are promising avenues to reduce unnecessary antibiotic use,[28] but caution is warranted in interpreting abnormal laboratory values in the absence of clinical signs. Follow-up radiographs may help differentiate pneumonia from retained lung fluid or surfactant deficiency and allow discontinuation of antibiotic therapy.[29] Once pneumonia is confirmed, there are limited clinical trials evaluating the optimal duration of therapy. One study suggests that 4 days of therapy may be sufficient in infants who are 35 or more weeks' gestation who are asymptomatic by 48 hours of antibiotic therapy.[30] Further trials are needed to determine the appropriate duration of therapy for preterm infants with pneumonia. Similarly, there is a paucity of treatment-duration studies on NEC, despite the higher inter-rater reliability of the Bell diagnostic criteria.[31,32] Given the relative frequency of these conditions, multicenter trials to determine appropriate treatment durations are feasible and warranted.

Maternal Chorioamnionitis

Another clinical situation leading to a high volume of antibiotic use is the management of infants born to mothers with chorioamnionitis. Although chorioamnionitis is a clear risk factor for neonatal sepsis, the current recommendation for obtaining a complete blood count and a blood culture and starting empiric antibiotic therapy was developed before the widespread use of IAP.[23,33] It remains unclear whether a laboratory evaluation with initiation of empiric therapy is warranted in well-appearing infants born to mothers with chorioamnionitis.[34,35] Because up to 4% of pregnancies are complicated by chorioamnionitis, upwards of 150,000 infants a year in the United States will receive empiric antibiotic therapy that many providers view as controversial. Further data are needed to determine how at risk well-appearing infants are if the mother received appropriate intrapartum antibiotic therapy.

Dosing and Therapeutic Drug Monitoring

Dosing and therapeutic monitoring of antimicrobials in neonates can be difficult. Neonates have both reduced glomerular filtration and tubular secretion compared with older children, and hepatic metabolic activity may vary extensively between preterm and term infants.[36] Even the ideal dosing strategy for vancomycin, an antibiotic invented more than 50 years ago, is unknown in neonates. In 2009, the Infectious Diseases Society of America (IDSA) and the American Society of Health-System Pharmacists recommended serum vancomycin troughs of 15 to 20 mg/L for the treatment of complicated methicillin-resistant *Staphylococcus aureus* infections (eg, bacteremia, meningitis) in adults.[37] Although studies have demonstrated the need for initial dosages between 60 and 70 mg/kg/d in hospitalized children,[38–40] none of these studies included infants less than 2 months of age. Monitoring of therapeutic drug levels can be limited because of concerns of iatrogenic blood loss, which may require red blood cell transfusions, particularly in low birth weight infants.[41]

Perioperative Prophylaxis

There is a significant knowledge gap regarding the optimal use of perioperative antibiotic prophylaxis for neonates. There are guidelines recommending one antibiotic agent for no more than 24 hours, or 48 hours for cardiac surgery; but these recommendations have not been extended to neonates.[42,43] Therefore, many infants continue to receive prolonged perioperative antibiotic prophylaxis, sometimes with multiple agents.[44,45] For abdominal wall defects, such as gastroschisis or omphalocele, some surgeons recommend antibiotic prophylaxis until closure, which is often delayed.[46] Even less is known regarding the optimal approach to infants undergoing extracorporeal membranous oxygenation (ECMO); a recent survey of ECMO centers revealed tremendous variation in the use of antibiotic prophylaxis before or during cannulation as well as in the antibiotics used and the duration of prophylaxis.[47] This variation is concerning as there is evidence that prolonged perioperative antibiotics do not prevent surgical site infections but may increase the risk of drug-resistant infections.[48,49]

ESSENTIAL PARTICIPANTS
The Antimicrobial Stewardship Team

In their 2007 guidelines, The IDSA and the Pediatric Infectious Diseases Society of America recommended creation of a multidisciplinary, interprofessional antimicrobial stewardship team for developing and implementing interventions in health care institutions.[50] Although the members may vary by the size and resources of the institution, the authors recommend that key members of the NICU antibiotic stewardship team should include a neonatologist, an infectious diseases (ID) physician, a neonatal or ID–trained pharmacist, infection preventionists, a bioinformatician, and a neonatal nurse. At smaller community hospitals, at minimum the stewardship team should consist of a neonatologist or hospitalist to lead stewardship interventions, a pharmacist to assist in neonatal dosing and drug monitoring, and a nurse or nurse practitioner for education and implementation.

Role of the Neonatologist

When few guidelines exist to guide antibiotic use, clinicians may be more likely to be influenced by institutional protocols or their fellow neonatologists.[51] Neonatologists may be more receptive to implementing changes in their practice if advocated by a well-respected peer rather than ID doctors or pharmacists. The neonatologist on the antibiotic stewardship team can help determine which stewardship metrics are meaningful to their peers and which interventions are preferred. He or she can coordinate with the NICU leadership to present data at division meetings and conferences. Ultimately, for stewardship efforts to be sustained, a paradigm shift is necessary from an ID physician restricting antibiotic use to the NICU and stewardship teams leading efforts to improve antibiotic use. This point is especially true in resource-limited settings, where the stewardship ID physician has other responsibilities, such as clinical care and infection control.

Other Participants

A bioinformatician can build computerized order entry tools that include dosing recommendations for gestational age and updated chronologic age and weight. Alerts can be created for renal dysfunction, trends in inflammatory markers, and cultures positive for MDROs.[52] Neonatal nurses regularly identify subtle symptoms or vital sign changes that indicate a new-onset infection or adverse events while on antibiotic therapy. Communication with the neonatal nurse is critical to determine whether the infants' clinical changes are isolated and potentially related to noninfectious causes or are persistent or worsening, suggesting a new or evolving infection. Antibiotic stewardship policies, particularly those involving the collection of diagnostic blood cultures or other blood samples, should, therefore, involve nurses' input. Microbiologists can assist in the review of institutional clinical microbiological data to guide empiric antibiotic recommendations for pathogens specific to the NICU.

MANAGEMENT STRATEGIES

A comprehensive approach to antibiotic use in the NICU, including accurate measurement of antibiotic use, improvement in diagnostic techniques, rational selection of empiric therapy, and continual re-evaluation and de-escalation or discontinuation when appropriate, is imperative to optimize clinical outcomes while minimizing the unintended consequences of antibiotic therapy.[50]

Measuring Antibiotic Use

Accurate measurement of antibiotic utilization is vital to identify targets of antibiotic stewardship, establish utilization benchmarks amongst institutions, and measure progress of stewardship interventions. Days of therapy (DOTs) is a commonly used metric in pediatrics and reflects total days of antimicrobial therapy administered, irrespective of dosing by weight or renal function.[50,53–55] DOTs are often adjusted for 1000 patient-days of hospitalization allowing benchmarking between children's hospitals.[56] Some considerations must be kept in mind when measuring antibiotic use with DOTs in the NICU setting. First, preterm infants may receive antibiotics in intervals less frequently than every 24 hours (eg, gentamicin may be administered as infrequently as every 48 hours); thus, DOTs may underestimate true antibiotic exposure. Second, preterm infants are likely to require prolonged hospitalization for nutritional support, with a decreasing requirement for antibiotic use as they approach term weight. Thus, the use of patient-days as a denominator to compare DOTs between institutions may be difficult if the proportions of preterm infants differ substantially. Finally, DOTs cannot measure antibiotic use at referring institutions. Although this is a general limitation with antibiotic stewardship metrics, it is particularly relevant for free-standing children's hospitals where most infants may be transferred from other institutions. **Table 2** lists potential antibiotic stewardship metrics for the NICU.

Adjudicating Antibiotic Use

The measurement of appropriate and inappropriate antibiotic use should be practical and useful to the prescribing neonatologists and should use institutional data when possible. Although some stewardship interventions are readily agreed on between the AS team and prescribing neonatologists (eg, targeting MDROs effectively), others such as the interpretation of colonization versus true infection and duration of treatment may be more difficult. For areas of disagreement, an initial first step could be to educate the NICU team on their own prescribing practices (eg, variation in the duration of culture-negative sepsis) to engender a discussion on best practice. It must be kept in mind that rotating on-service neonatologists have different durations of service time; thus, assigning individual responsibility for specific antimicrobial usage may not be possible. Thus, the presentation of the prescribing data as a team effort may be

Table 2
Useful antimicrobial stewardship metrics for the NICU

Primary Drivers	Secondary Drivers	Metrics
Avoid redundant antibiotic use	Reduce concurrent use of antibiotics with anaerobic spectrum of activity	DOT of concurrent use of piperacillin-tazobactam, meropenem, or imipenem with metronidazole >1 d
Reduce broad spectrum antibiotic use	Reduce use of broad-spectrum perioperative antibiotic prophylaxis for clean surgical procedures	DOT of noncefazolin perioperative prophylaxis for cardiac surgery
	Reduce use of vancomycin	DOT vancomycin
	Reduce use of third-generation cephalosporins	DOT third-generation cephalosporins
Reduce duration of antibiotic use	Avoid prolonged duration of postoperative prophylaxis	DOT of perioperative prophylaxis >48 h
	Avoid prolonged duration of culture-negative sepsis	Interquartile range of DOTs for duration of culture-negative sepsis
Avoid inadequate therapy	Reduce episodes of bug-drug mismatch for treatment of late-onset sepsis	DOT of inadequate therapy per 100 LOS evaluations

most useful.[57] Institutional clinical microbiology data should be used to guide the selection of empiric antibiotic therapy. Although the creation of NICU-specific antibiograms may not be possible because of a limited number of infections per genera, instances of a bug-drug mismatch can help determine if existing practices need to be altered. If possible, stratification by age younger than 7 days versus older than 7 days would be helpful as the pathogens and empiric antibiotic regimens differ between these 2 groups.[58] **Table 3** lists possible stewardship interventions.

Maximizing Culture Yields

Procurement of adequate volume of blood for cultures can improve sensitivity. In clinical studies, most infants with sepsis have well more than 5 colony-forming units (CFU) per milliliter in their blood; up to 33% may have more than 1000 CFU/mL.[59] Schelonka

Table 3
Suggestions for stewardship in the NICU

Strategy	Examples of Stewardship
Diagnosis	Institutional guidelines for obtaining and interpreting respiratory tract cultures, to avoid treatment of colonization
Empiric therapy	Develop NICU-specific antibiograms for Gram-negative infections as a group
Dose optimization	Use automated pharmacy alerts to identify infants who are receiving inadequate dosing for suspected meningitis
Prescriber audit and feedback	Use prospective audit and feedback to identify opportunities to target pathogens in infants with positive cultures
Duration of therapy	Establish institutional protocols for the duration of treatment of NEC and culture-negative sepsis

and colleagues[60] demonstrated that inoculation of 1 mL of blood could detect neonatal pathogens at blood concentrations as low as 4 CFU/mL. The most recent American Academy of Pediatrics' guidelines on the management of neonates with suspected sepsis recommend obtaining a minimum of 1 mL of blood for culture when sepsis is suspected.[61] Audits of blood cultures obtained from NICUs show that the median volume is often less than 1 mL but can be improved with education of the providers responsible for the blood draw.[62,63] Finally, cultures obtained from nonsterile sites, including endotracheal tubes, should be interpreted with caution to avoid treatment of colonization rather than infection.[64]

Ancillary Laboratory Tests

In the absence of a test with sufficient sensitivity to prevent the initiation of antibiotic therapy, investigators have focused on non–culture-based diagnostics as a supplement to culture.[65] The complete blood count and differential has been used in sepsis evaluations for decades,[66] and the negative predictive value of serially normal immature-to-total neutrophil ratios approaches 100% when the blood cultures are sterile.[67] However, the positive predictive value of serial blood counts is poor. Other evaluated biomarkers include C-reactive protein, procalcitonin, and cytokines, such as interleukins 6 and 8. There has been increased interest in developing risk-prediction models that may allow clinicians to withhold antibiotics in the lowest-risk infants, but these models have not been evaluated rigorously and may lack the sensitivity needed for clinicians to feel comfortable withholding antibiotic therapy.[68,69] Heart rate monitoring as a physiologic predictor of impending sepsis shows promise, although what its effect on antibiotic stewardship will be is unclear.[70] In general, these biomarkers may be able to improve the negative predictive value of a sterile culture; their use in combination with appropriate blood cultures can lead to reduced antibiotic use.[71,72] The improved accessibility and speed of these tests, including their availability on a point-of-care microarray, may increase their clinical utility and allow further studies on their impact on antibiotic stewardship.[73] Although promising, these tests are at present ancillary at best to appropriately drawn cultures.[74] Making antibiotic decisions based on properly obtained cultures will help to decrease unnecessary or prolonged antibiotic therapy.[22]

Choosing Empiric Therapy

Once appropriate cultures are obtained, empiric therapy that covers the most likely pathogens should be initiated. Group B *Streptococcus* and Enterobacteriaceae, such as *Escherichia coli*, remain the most common causes of EOS (<7 days of age); other Gram-negative bacilli, *Candida spp*, and *Staphylococcus* are additional causes of LOS.[75,76] A combination of ampicillin and gentamicin remain the appropriate therapy for EOS, despite the increase in ampicillin-resistant pathogens.[61] Third-generation cephalosporins should be avoided in the absence of meningitis because of concerns for resistance and increased rates of invasive candidiasis, particularly in low birth weight infants.[4,5]

Appropriate empiric therapy for LOS includes a semisynthetic penicillin, such as oxacillin or nafcillin, in combination with an aminoglycoside. Alternatively, piperacillin-tazobactam or cefepime can be used for Gram-negative coverage, especially in infants known to be colonized with resistant Gram-negative organisms. Whether these agents are associated with increased rates of invasive candidiasis has not been well studied. Third-generation cephalosporins are best reserved for cases when meningitis is suspected. Coagulase-negative *Staphylococcus* (CoNS) is not routinely covered by oxacillin or nafcillin, but there is evidence suggesting that

CoNS infection is not associated with increased mortality.[77] Therefore, some units have implemented vancomycin-reduction guidelines (**Box 1**) that reserve vancomycin use for infants with persistent CoNS bacteremia or those with methicillin-resistant *Staphylococcus aureus* infection.[78]

Reevaluating Antibiotic Use Once Initiated

Using the culture results and the infant's clinical course, providers should continually review the initial antibiotic regimen. Antibiotics should be discontinued if the cultures remain sterile by 48 hours, provided the infant is improved.[61] If a pathogen is recovered, antibiotics should be changed to the narrowest-spectrum agent that has activity against the pathogen and distributes to the infected body site. Failure to narrow or de-escalate therapy based on culture results is one of the most common causes of inappropriate antibiotic use in the NICU.[79] An electronic medical record hard stop is an effective means of reducing inadvertent use of antibiotics beyond 48 hours of sterile cultures.[80]

Box 1
Vancomycin reduction guideline

For infants more than 3 days of age with suspected late-onset sepsis, provided that they are not known or suspected to be colonized with methicillin-resistant *Staphylococcus aureus*

1. Obtain blood cultures and consider obtaining cerebrospinal fluid (CSF) culture; obtain adjunctive diagnostic markers (complete blood count with differential, C-reactive protein) at provider discretion

2. Begin therapy with oxacillin (or nafcillin) and gentamicin

3. If the initial cultures are sterile at 48 hours

   a. Consider discontinuing antibiotic therapy.

   b. If the infant is clinically improved and the provider thinks that continued therapy is warranted, continue the current therapy.

   c. If the infant is deteriorating, obtain a second set of blood cultures and consider changing to vancomycin and gentamicin empirically.

   d. If the second set of blood cultures is sterile at 48 hours, again consider discontinuing antibiotic therapy.

4. If the initial cultures grow oxacillin-resistant coagulase-negative *Staphylococcus*

   a. Draw a second set of blood cultures, obtain CSF culture if not already collected, and change antibiotic therapy to vancomycin alone. The clinical scenario should guide the duration of therapy.

   b. If the second set of cultures is sterile at 48 hours, consider discontinuing all antibiotics on the basis that initial cultures may represent contamination.

   c. If the second set of cultures also grow oxacillin-resistant coagulase-negative *Staphylococcus*

      i. Verify with microbiology that they are the same species.

      ii. Continue therapy with vancomycin.

      iii. Consider removing indwelling catheters.

Adapted from Chiu CH, Michelow IC, Cronin J, et al. Effectiveness of a guideline to reduce vancomycin use in the neonatal intensive care unit. Pediatr Infect Dis J 2011;30:275; with permission.

AREAS WHERE MORE WORK IS NEEDED

Coordinating Stewardship with Obstetricians

Collaborations with obstetricians are necessary to reduce antibiotic exposure in the perinatal period. Failure to follow antibiotic prophylaxis recommendations during pregnancy may lead to an unnecessary empiric antibiotic during evaluations for sepsis in neonates.[81] This practice is particularly concerning for preterm infants as their mothers are less likely to receive IAP than mothers of term infants.[82] Even when IAP is initiated, guidelines for the selection of IAP may not be followed. For example, despite the recommendation that pregnant women with penicillin allergies at low risk for anaphylaxis receive cefazolin for IAP,[23] Van Dyke and colleagues[82] demonstrated that women were more likely to receive clindamycin (70%) than cefazolin (14%), a more efficacious agent. Approximately 15% of invasive group B *streptococcus* isolates in the United States are resistant to clindamycin.[83]

Organizing with Other NICU Quality Efforts

The most important measures to decrease antibiotic use in the NICU may be preventative. Prevention of preterm delivery logically will decrease the amount of antibiotic administered to preterm infants. Administration of progesterone to mothers at risk for recurrent preterm delivery is an encouraging strategy that is currently being evaluated further.[84] Within the NICU, adherence to infection-prevention strategies, including hand hygiene and appropriate central line care, will limit horizontal transmission of infectious agents.

Building a Research Infrastructure

Generalizable metrics of antibiotic utilization, readily obtainable from the electronic health record, are necessary for benchmarking between institutions. Multicenter collaborations can provide the number of patients needed to conduct comparative effectiveness studies. Large neonatal clinical databases can be used for comparative effectiveness research.[85] Possible areas of investigation include the brief versus prolonged perioperative prophylaxis for prevention of surgical site infections following cardiac surgery, comparison of antimicrobial regimens for the treatment of NEC, and comparison of agents and durations of therapy for EOS and LOS. Reports of adverse events with new antimicrobials can be shared between centers. Pooling of microbiological data can be used to create NICU-specific regional and national antibiograms to guide empiric therapy.

SUMMARY

Neonatologists care for a population at high risk for sepsis who present with very nonspecific signs. Neonates often receive prolonged antibiotic therapy for treatment of culture-negative sepsis. Multidisciplinary collaboration and meaningful antibiotic stewardship metrics for neonatologists are necessary. Key stewardship interventions include collection of appropriate blood cultures, use of ancillary laboratory tests, avoidance of unnecessarily broad empiric therapy, and de-escalation or discontinuation of therapy. Future efforts should include coordinating with other quality-improvement efforts and building a national research infrastructure.

REFERENCES

1. Clark RH, Bloom BT, Spitzer AR, et al. Reported medication use in the neonatal intensive care unit: data from a large national data set. Pediatrics 2006;117:1979–87.

2. Lesch CA, Itokazu GS, Danziger LH, et al. Multi-hospital analysis of antimicrobial usage and resistance trends. Diagn Microbiol Infect Dis 2001;41:149–54.
3. Singh N, Patel KM, Leger MM, et al. Risk of resistant infections with Enterobacteriaceae in hospitalized neonates. Pediatr Infect Dis J 2002;21:1029–33.
4. de Man P, Verhoeven BA, Verbrugh HA, et al. An antibiotic policy to prevent emergence of resistant bacilli. Lancet 2000;355:973–8.
5. Cotten CM, McDonald S, Stoll B, et al. The association of third-generation cephalosporin use and invasive candidiasis in extremely low birth-weight infants. Pediatrics 2006;118:717–22.
6. Lee JH, Hornik CP, Benjamin DK Jr, et al. Risk factors for invasive candidiasis in infants >1500 g birth weight. Pediatr Infect Dis J 2013;32:222–6.
7. Saiman L, Ludington E, Dawson JD, et al. Risk factors for Candida species colonization of neonatal intensive care unit patients. Pediatr Infect Dis J 2001;20: 1119–24.
8. Cotten CM, Taylor S, Stoll B, et al. Prolonged duration of initial empirical antibiotic treatment is associated with increased rates of necrotizing enterocolitis and death for extremely low birth weight infants. Pediatrics 2009;123:58–66.
9. Kuppala VS, Meinzen-Derr J, Morrow AL, et al. Prolonged initial empirical antibiotic treatment is associated with adverse outcomes in premature infants. J Pediatr 2011;159:720–5.
10. Alexander VN, Northrup V, Bizzarro MJ. Antibiotic exposure in the newborn intensive care unit and the risk of necrotizing enterocolitis. J Pediatr 2011;159: 392–7.
11. Torrazza RM, Neu J. The altered gut microbiome and necrotizing enterocolitis. Clin Perinatol 2013;40:93–108.
12. Wang Y, Hoenig JD, Malin KJ, et al. 16S rRNA gene-based analysis of fecal microbiota from preterm infants with and without necrotizing enterocolitis. ISME J 2009;3:944–54.
13. Ferraris L, Butel MJ, Campeotto F, et al. Clostridia in premature neonates' gut: incidence, antibiotic susceptibility, and perinatal determinants influencing colonization. PLoS One 2012;7:e30594.
14. Valles Y, Gosalbes MJ, de Vries LE, et al. Metagenomics and development of the gut microbiota in infants. Clin Microbiol Infect 2012;18(Suppl 4):21–6.
15. Goldstein EJ. Beyond the target pathogen: ecological effects of the hospital formulary. Curr Opin Infect Dis 2011;24(Suppl 1):S21–31.
16. Fischer JE. Physicians' ability to diagnose sepsis in newborns and critically ill children. Pediatr Crit Care Med 2005;6:S120–5.
17. Ottolini MC, Lundgren K, Mirkinson LJ, et al. Utility of complete blood count and blood culture screening to diagnose neonatal sepsis in the asymptomatic at risk newborn. Pediatr Infect Dis J 2003;22:430–4.
18. Bekhof J, Reitsma JB, Kok JH, et al. Clinical signs to identify late-onset sepsis in preterm infants. Eur J Pediatr 2013;172:501–8.
19. Shani L, Weitzman D, Melamed R, et al. Risk factors for early sepsis in very low birth weight neonates with respiratory distress syndrome. Acta Paediatr 2008; 97:12–5.
20. Weintraub AS, Cadet CT, Perez R, et al. Antibiotic use in newborns with transient tachypnea of the newborn. Neonatology 2013;103:235–40.
21. Dempsey EM, Barrington KJ. Diagnostic criteria and therapeutic interventions for the hypotensive very low birth weight infant. J Perinatol 2006;26:677–81.
22. Cantey JB, Sanchez PJ. Prolonged antibiotic therapy for "culture-negative" sepsis in preterm infants: it's time to stop! J Pediatr 2011;159:707–8.

23. Verani JR, McGee L, Schrag SJ, Division of Bacterial Diseases, National Center for Immunization and Respiratory Diseases, Centers for Disease Control and Prevention (CDC). Prevention of perinatal group B streptococcal disease–revised guidelines from CDC, 2010. MMWR Recomm Rep 2010;59:1–36.

24. Cordero L, Ayers LW. Duration of empiric antibiotics for suspected early-onset sepsis in extremely low birth weight infants. Infect Control Hosp Epidemiol 2003;24:662–6.

25. Manktelow BN, Draper ES, Field DJ. Predicting neonatal mortality among very preterm infants: a comparison of three versions of the CRIB score. Arch Dis Child Fetal Neonatal Ed 2010;95:F9–13.

26. Spitzer AR, Kirkby S, Kornhauser M. Practice variation in suspected neonatal sepsis: a costly problem in neonatal intensive care. J Perinatol 2005;25:265–9.

27. Liem TB, Krediet TG, Fleer A, et al. Variation in antibiotic use in neonatal intensive care units in the Netherlands. J Antimicrob Chemother 2010;65:1270–5.

28. Pinto MC, Bueno AC, Vieira AA. Implementation of a protocol for antibiotic use in very low birth weight infants. J Pediatr (Rio J) 2013;89(5):450–5.

29. Haney PJ, Bohlman M, Sun CC. Radiographic findings in neonatal pneumonia. AJR Am J Roentgenol 1984;143:23–6.

30. Engle WD, Jackson GL, Sendelbach D, et al. Neonatal pneumonia: comparison of 4 vs 7 days of antibiotic therapy in term and near-term infants. J Perinatol 2000;20:421–6.

31. Neu J. Necrotizing enterocolitis: the search for a unifying pathogenic theory leading to prevention. Pediatr Clin North Am 1996;43:409–32.

32. Downard CD, Renaud E, St Peter SD, et al. Treatment of necrotizing enterocolitis: an American Pediatric Surgical Association Outcomes and Clinical Trials Committee systematic review. J Pediatr Surg 2012;47:2111–22.

33. Lieberman E, Lang J, Richardson DK, et al. Intrapartum maternal fever and neonatal outcome. Pediatrics 2000;105:8–13.

34. Linder N, Fridman E, Makhoul A, et al. Management of term newborns following maternal intrapartum fever. J Matern Fetal Neonatal Med 2013;26:207–10.

35. Taylor JA, Opel DJ. Choriophobia: a 1-act play. Pediatrics 2012;130:342–6.

36. Koren G. Therapeutic drug monitoring principles in the neonate. National Academy of Clinical Biochemistry. Clin Chem 1997;43:222–7.

37. Rybak M, Lomaestro B, Rotschafer JC, et al. Therapeutic monitoring of vancomycin in adult patients: a consensus review of the American Society of Health-System Pharmacists, the Infectious Diseases Society of America, and the Society of Infectious Diseases Pharmacists. Am J Health Syst Pharm 2009;66:82–98.

38. Le J, Bradley JS, Murray W, et al. Improved vancomycin dosing in children using area under the curve exposure. Pediatr Infect Dis J 2013;32:e155–63.

39. Chhim RF, Arnold SR, Lee KR. Vancomycin dosing practices, trough concentrations, and predicted area under the curve in children with suspected invasive Staphylococcal infections. J Pediatric Infect Dis Soc 2013;2:259–62.

40. Demirjian A, Finkelstein Y, Nava-Ocampo A, et al. A randomized controlled trial of a vancomycin loading dose in children. Pediatr Infect Dis J 2013;32:1217–23.

41. Widness JA. Pathophysiology of anemia during the neonatal period, including anemia of prematurity. Neoreviews 2008;9:e520.

42. Bratzler DW, Hunt DR. The surgical infection prevention and surgical care improvement projects: national initiatives to improve outcomes for patients having surgery. Clin Infect Dis 2006;43:322–30.

43. Berenguer CM, Ochsner MG Jr, Lord SA, et al. Improving surgical site infections: using National Surgical Quality Improvement Program data to institute

Surgical Care Improvement Project protocols in improving surgical outcomes. J Am Coll Surg 2010;210:737–41, 41–3.

44. Amadeo B, Zarb P, Muller A, et al. European Surveillance of Antibiotic Consumption (ESAC) point prevalence survey 2008: paediatric antimicrobial prescribing in 32 hospitals of 21 European countries. J Antimicrob Chemother 2010;65: 2247–52.

45. Alphonso N, Anagnostopoulos PV, Scarpace S, et al. Perioperative antibiotic prophylaxis in paediatric cardiac surgery. Cardiol Young 2007;17:12–25.

46. Baird R, Puligandla P, Skarsgard E, et al, Canadian Pediatric Surgical Network. Infectious complications in the management of gastroschisis. Pediatr Surg Int 2012;28:399–404.

47. Kao LS, Fleming GM, Escamilla RJ, et al. Antimicrobial prophylaxis and infection surveillance in extracorporeal membrane oxygenation patients: a multi-institutional survey of practice patterns. ASAIO J 2011;57:231–8.

48. Alvarez P, Fuentes C, Garcia N, et al. Evaluation of the duration of the antibiotic prophylaxis in paediatric postoperative heart surgery patients. Pediatr Cardiol 2012;33:735–8.

49. Knoderer CA, Cox EG, Berg MD, et al. Efficacy of limited cefuroxime prophylaxis in pediatric patients after cardiovascular surgery. Am J Health Syst Pharm 2011; 68:909–14.

50. Dellit TH, Owens RC, McGowan JE Jr, et al. Infectious Diseases Society of America and the Society for Healthcare Epidemiology of America guidelines for developing an institutional program to enhance antimicrobial stewardship. Clin Infect Dis 2007;44:159–77.

51. Patel S, Landers T, Larson E, et al. Clinical vignettes provide an understanding of antibiotic prescribing practices in neonatal intensive care units. Infect Control Hosp Epidemiol 2011;32:597–602.

52. Sheehan B, Chused A, Graham PL 3rd, et al. Frequency and types of alerts for antibiotic prescribing in a neonatal ICU. Stud Health Technol Inform 2009;146: 521–5.

53. Valcourt K, Norozian F, Lee H, et al. Drug use density in critically ill children and newborns: analysis of various methodologies. Pediatr Crit Care Med 2009;10: 495–9.

54. Polk RE, Fox C, Mahoney A, et al. Measurement of adult antibacterial drug use in 130 US hospitals: comparison of defined daily dose and days of therapy. Clin Infect Dis 2007;44:664–70.

55. Centers for Disease Control and Prevention. Antimicrobial use and resistance module. Atlanta (GA): CDC; 2013.

56. Gerber JS, Newland JG, Coffin SE, et al. Variability in antibiotic use at children's hospitals. Pediatrics 2010;126:1067–73.

57. Patel SJ, Saiman L, Duchon JM, et al. Development of an antimicrobial stewardship intervention using a model of actionable feedback. Interdiscip Perspect Infect Dis 2012;2012:150367.

58. Tamma PD, Robinson GL, Gerber JS, et al. Pediatric antimicrobial susceptibility trends across the United States. Infect Control Hosp Epidemiol 2013;34:1244–51.

59. Dietzman DE, Fischer GW, Schoenknecht FD. Neonatal Escherichia coli septicemia–bacterial counts in blood. J Pediatr 1974;85:128–30.

60. Schelonka RL, Chai MK, Yoder BA, et al. Volume of blood required to detect common neonatal pathogens. J Pediatr 1996;129:275–8.

61. Polin RA, Committee on Fetus and Newborn. Management of neonates with suspected or proven early-onset bacterial sepsis. Pediatrics 2012;129:1006–15.

62. Connell TG, Rele M, Cowley D, et al. How reliable is a negative blood culture result? Volume of blood submitted for culture in routine practice in a children's hospital. Pediatrics 2007;119:891–6.

63. van Ingen J, Hilt N, Bosboom R. Education of phlebotomy teams improves blood volume in blood culture bottles. J Clin Microbiol 2013;51:1020–1.

64. Tamma PD, Turnbull AE, Milstone AM, et al. Ventilator-associated tracheitis in children: does antibiotic duration matter? Clin Infect Dis 2011;52:1324–31.

65. Malik A, Hui CP, Pennie RA, et al. Beyond the complete blood cell count and C-reactive protein: a systematic review of modern diagnostic tests for neonatal sepsis. Arch Pediatr Adolesc Med 2003;157:511–6.

66. Manroe BL, Weinberg AG, Rosenfeld CR, et al. The neonatal blood count in health and disease. I. Reference values for neutrophilic cells. J Pediatr 1979;95:89–98.

67. Murphy K, Weiner J. Use of leukocyte counts in evaluation of early-onset neonatal sepsis. Pediatr Infect Dis J 2012;31:16–9.

68. Puopolo KM, Escobar GJ. Early-onset sepsis: a predictive model based on maternal risk factors. Curr Opin Pediatr 2013;25:161–6.

69. Pinto MC, Bueno AC, Vieira AA. Implementation of a protocol proposed by the Brazilian National Health Surveillance Agency for antibiotic use in very low birth weight infants. J Pediatr (Rio J) 2013;89:450–5.

70. Fairchild KD, Schelonka RL, Kaufman DA, et al. Septicemia mortality reduction in neonates in a heart rate characteristics monitoring trial. Pediatr Res 2013; 74(5):570–5.

71. Franz AR, Bauer K, Schalk A, et al. Measurement of interleukin 8 in combination with C-reactive protein reduced unnecessary antibiotic therapy in newborn infants: a multicenter, randomized, controlled trial. Pediatrics 2004;114:1–8.

72. Hayashi Y, Paterson DL. Strategies for reduction in duration of antibiotic use in hospitalized patients. Clin Infect Dis 2011;52:1232–40.

73. Buchegger P, Sauer U, Toth-Szekely H, et al. Miniaturized protein microarray with internal calibration as point-of-care device for diagnosis of neonatal sepsis. Sensors (Basel) 2012;12:1494–508.

74. Camacho-Gonzalez A, Spearman PW, Stoll BJ. Neonatal infectious diseases: evaluation of neonatal sepsis. Pediatr Clin North Am 2013;60:367–89.

75. Stoll BJ, Hansen NI, Sanchez PJ, et al. Early onset neonatal sepsis: the burden of group B Streptococcal and E. coli disease continues. Pediatrics 2011;127: 817–26.

76. Stoll BJ, Hansen N, Fanaroff AA, et al. Late-onset sepsis in very low birth weight neonates: the experience of the NICHD Neonatal Research Network. Pediatrics 2002;110:285–91.

77. Karlowicz MG, Buescher ES, Surka AE. Fulminant late-onset sepsis in a neonatal intensive care unit, 1988-1997, and the impact of avoiding empiric vancomycin therapy. Pediatrics 2000;106:1387–90.

78. Chiu CH, Michelow IC, Cronin J, et al. Effectiveness of a guideline to reduce vancomycin use in the neonatal intensive care unit. Pediatr Infect Dis J 2011; 30:273–8.

79. Patel SJ, Oshodi A, Prasad P, et al. Antibiotic use in neonatal intensive care units and adherence with Centers for Disease Control and Prevention 12 Step Campaign to Prevent Antimicrobial Resistance. Pediatr Infect Dis J 2009;28: 1047–51.

80. Jardine MA, Kumar Y, Kausalya S, et al. Reducing antibiotic use on the neonatal unit by improving communication of blood culture results: a completed audit cycle. Arch Dis Child Fetal Neonatal Ed 2003;88:F255.

81. Tripathi N, Cotten CM, Smith PB. Antibiotic use and misuse in the neonatal intensive care unit. Clin Perinatol 2012;39:61–8.

82. Van Dyke MK, Phares CR, Lynfield R, et al. Evaluation of universal antenatal screening for group B streptococcus. N Engl J Med 2009;360:2626–36.

83. Phares CR, Lynfield R, Farley MM, et al. Epidemiology of invasive group B streptococcal disease in the United States, 1999-2005. JAMA 2008;299:2056–65.

84. Dodd JM, Jones L, Flenady V, et al. Prenatal administration of progesterone for preventing preterm birth in women considered to be at risk of preterm birth. Cochrane Database Syst Rev 2013;(7):CD004947.

85. Pediatrix Medical Group's Clinical Data Warehouse (CDW) fact sheet. 2013. Available: http://www.pediatrix.com/sitemaker/websitefiles/PDX52475423/workfiles/newsroom/CDW%20Fact%20Sheet%204.3.12.pdf. Accessed November 9, 2013.

Antimicrobial Stewardship in Immunocompromised Hosts

Lilian M. Abbo, MD[a],*, Ella J. Ariza-Heredia, MD[b]

KEYWORDS

- Antimicrobial stewardship • Transplant • Solid organ • Hematologic malignancies
- Neutropenia • Fever • Immunocompromised

KEY POINTS

- Immunocompromised hosts are increasingly colonized and infected by multidrug-resistant organisms with limited antimicrobial treatment options.
- Implementation of antimicrobial stewardship strategies in immunocompromised hosts is challenging, but there are multiple opportunities to improve the selection, dosing, and duration of antimicrobial agents.
- Collaboration with local experts, such as oncologists and transplant teams, is fundamental for a successful stewardship program for the immunocompromised population.
- The use of early and appropriate diagnostic testing is essential to guide therapy and minimize nonessential antimicrobial exposure.

INTRODUCTION

For decades, infections have constituted a major threat for patients with febrile neutropenia,[1,2] solid organ transplant (SOT),[3] and hematopoietic stem cell transplantation (HSCT).[4] It is well recognized that the diagnosis and treatment of infections in immunocompromised hosts is more difficult than in persons with normal immune function. The spectrum of potential pathogens is broad, infection often progresses rapidly, and invasive diagnostic procedures are often required for accurate and timely diagnosis.[5] Early and specific microbiologic diagnosis in immunocompromised hosts is essential for guiding treatment and minimizing nonessential antimicrobial therapy with potential serious adverse reactions as well as possible interactions with immunosuppressive agents.[3,4]

Over the past few decades, there has been a dramatic reduction in the development of antimicrobial agents with novel mechanisms of action to combat the rising spread of

Disclosures: The authors have nothing to disclose.
[a] Division of Infectious Diseases, Department of Medicine, University of Miami Miller School of Medicine, 1120 Northwest 14th Street, Suite 851, Miami, FL 33136, USA; [b] Division of Infectious Diseases, Department of Internal Medicine, The University of Texas MD Anderson Cancer Center, 1515 Holcombe Boulevard, Unit 1460, Houston, TX 77030, USA
* Corresponding author.
E-mail address: labbo@med.miami.edu

infections caused by antimicrobial multidrug-resistant organisms (MDROs).[6] MDROs are an emerging threat in high-risk immunocompromised hosts, such as SOT and HSCT recipients, and those with hematologic malignancies exposed to cytotoxic chemotherapy and prolonged neutropenia. Although it has long been recognized that these patients are among the highest risk for becoming colonized and developing serious infections, the frequency with which MDROs cause infection in these recipients has increased significantly in the past several years.[7-9]

Numerous studies have been published demonstrating that antimicrobial resistance has an adverse impact on patient safety and quality of care.[10-13] As a result, there is increasing awareness about the importance of judicious use of antimicrobials, or antimicrobial stewardship. To date, there are no antimicrobial stewardship guidelines focusing on high-risk immunocompromised hosts.[14] Appropriate management of antimicrobials in these patients is important but challenging.[15] Furthermore, confirming the presence of infection can be difficult and the diagnostic uncertainty contributes to the use of broad-spectrum antimicrobials for extended periods of time. Other important challenges are the perceptions and behaviors regarding antimicrobial use by multiple physicians caring for these patients. Barriers to the implementation of antimicrobial stewardship strategies in immunocompromised hosts are summarized in **Box 1**. This article focuses on the challenges, opportunities, and areas for further study in the implementation of successful antimicrobial stewardship strategies in high-risk immunocompromised hosts.

GOALS OF ANTIMICROBIAL STEWARDSHIP IN IMMUNOCOMPROMISED HOSTS

Antimicrobial stewardship programs (ASPs) aim to optimize the appropriate selection, dosing, route, and duration of antimicrobial therapy while limiting unintended consequences, such as the emergence of resistance, adverse drug events, and cost.[16] These goals are relevant for immunosuppressed patients because infections have constituted a major threat to the success of transplantation for many decades and

---

Box 1
Challenges to the implementation of antimicrobial stewardship in immunocompromised hosts

1. Physician perceptions and attitudes—"my patient is sicker than yours"
2. Wide range of possible infectious etiologies with diagnostic uncertainty
3. Impaired inflammatory responses
4. Difficulty in making an early diagnosis
5. Urgency for empiric effective antimicrobial therapy
6. Significant drug toxicities and potent drug interactions
7. Prolonged exposure to prophylactic antibiotics may lead to antimicrobial resistance
8. Increasing antimicrobial resistance with limited therapeutic options to appropriately treat empirically or documented infections
9. Difficulty with distinguishing rejection and graft versus host disease from infections
10. Difficulty in controlling the source of infection due to issues, such as thrombocytopenia, limiting surgical interventions
11. Prolonged duration of immunosuppressed state increases the risk for uncommon presentations of common and uncommon infections
12. Duration of antimicrobial therapy not clearly defined in many infections for these patients

are one of the leading causes of morbidity and mortality in febrile neutropenia, after SOT and HSCT.[3,10] Given the need for both prevention and treatment of infections in immunocompromised patients, antimicrobials are commonly used for prolonged periods of time leading to significant changes in a patient's normal endogenous micro-biota.[15] These changes increase the risk for colonization and infection with MDROs and *Clostridium difficile*.[17] ASPs help clinicians tailor these prophylactic and treatment regimens according to clinical risks, toxicities, and local patterns of antimicrobial resistance.

EMERGENCE OF ANTIMICROBIAL RESISTANCE IN IMMUNOCOMPROMISED HOSTS

Infections caused by multidrug-resistant gram-negative organisms in organ trans-plantation are of concern on a global scale, with increasing reports in at least 5 continents.[18–22] Cohorts from the United States and Spain have demonstrated that gram-negative bacteria represent the most commonly transmitted donor pathogen in SOT recipients.[18] Donor-derived infections with MDROs are frequently associated with resistance to commonly used prophylactic antibiotics, even in solid organ donors hospitalized for fewer than 6 days prior to organ procurement.[9] Several studies have described that delays in the selection of the optimal antimicrobial therapy could have a negative impact on survival from infectious caused by those organisms in organ re-cipients and often require the use of antimicrobials that are more toxic and less effec-tive than those used to treat susceptible pathogens.[23–25] Surveillance of local patterns of antimicrobial resistance in hematology-oncology and transplant centers should be carried out, with a review of the situation one or twice yearly, and a top 10 list of relevant pathogens should be defined.[26] These trends should serve as a guide to ASPs to develop specific pathways and policies in collaboration with primary care teams, for whether or not to use antibiotic prophylaxis in certain categories of patients, to determine the need and frequency of surveillance cultures to detect colo-nization, and to develop hospital-specific guidelines for prophylactic and empiric antimicrobials.[26,27]

Fluoroquinolone Prophylaxis

Fluoroquinolone prophylaxis is recommended as a consideration for patients with expected durations of profound and prolonged neutropenia (absolute neutrophil count ≤ 100 cells/mm^3 for greater than 7 days).[2] The widespread use of fluoroqui-nolones has likely contributed to a decline in their effectiveness as treatment op-tions as well as an increase in the prevalence of fluoroquinolone resistance.[28–30] Fluoroquinolone use has also been associated with higher risk for colonization and infection with methicillin-resistant *Staphylococcus aureus* (MRSA) in neutro-penic cancer patients and significantly increased risk for breakthrough bacteremia with multidrug-resistant *Enterobacteriaceae* and multidrug-resistant *Pseudomonas aeruginosa* (**Table 1**).[28,33,38,45] Although prophylaxis with quinolones exerts a signif-icant selection pressure for colonization and infection by fluoroquinolone-resistant organisms, a recent Cochrane review confirmed earlier meta-analyses that the reduction in mortality and infection rates in high-risk patients still outweighs the risk of resistance, the costs, and occasional adverse events.[46] Therefore, quinolone prophylaxis should be used only in selected high-risk patients, not in all neutropenic patients.[26]

Local patterns of resistance should be closely monitored. In settings with a high prevalence of quinolone resistance, these agents should be avoided as empiric mono-therapy in patients with presumptive infections.

Table 1
Increased risk of infection by antibiotic-resistant organisms with the use of fluoroquinolones

Organisms	References
Gram-positives	
MRSA	Graffunder & Venezia,[31] 2002 Campillo et al,[32] 2001 Weber et al,[33] 2003
VRE	Liu et al,[34] 2012 Bodro et al,[35] 2013
Streptococcus viridans	Prabhu et al,[36] 2005
Gram-negatives	
Fluoroquinolone-resistant *Pseudomonas* *aeruginosa* and *Enterobacteriaceae*	Yoo et al,[37] 1997 Rangaraj et al,[38] 2010
ESBL-producing *Escherichia coli* and *Klebsiella pneumoniae*	Lautenbach et al,[39] 2001 Paterson et al,[40] 2000 Garnica et al,[41] 2013
Other non-fermenting gram-negative organisms (*Acinetobacter spp, Stenotrophomonas*)	Irfan et al,[42] 2008
Anaerobes	
C difficile	Golledge et al,[43] 1992 Weiss,[44] 2009 Pepin et al,[29] 2005

Empiric Carbapenem Therapy

Carbapenem monotherapy is approved as empiric therapy for febrile neutropenic patients.[2] Nonetheless, judicious use of these agents is strongly encouraged considering the global increase of carbapenem-resistant Enterobactericeae (CRE), the limited therapeutic agents available to treat infections with MDROs, and a possible association between carbapenem use and a higher incidence of *C difficile* in neutropenic patients.[47,48] CRE are associated with potentially more toxic therapies and worse outcomes in transplant patients than in patients not infected with these resistant strains.[17,21] These organisms have become a significant global public health challenge but the optimal treatment remains undefined. Alternative antimicrobials, such as cefepime or piperacillin/tazobactam, are preferred in the empiric treatment of patients with fever and neutropenia.[47,48] Exceptions include patients with severe sepsis, septic shock, history of infections with extended-spectrum β-lactamase (ESBL)-producing organisms, or multidrug-resistant *Pseudomonas* while awaiting culture results. De-escalation should be considered if the infection has resolved, narrower therapeutic alternatives are available, or neutropenia has recovered.[49]

Empiric Vancomycin Therapy

Widespread vancomycin use has been associated with the spread of vancomycin-resistant enterococcus (VRE).[50] Bloodstream infections caused by VRE have been associated with prolonged duration of bacteremia and an independent risk for mortality in neutropenic patients compared with vancomycin susceptible infections.[51] A meta-analysis of 13 randomized trials assessed outcomes of febrile neutropenic patients receiving empiric glycopeptide therapy compared with patients not receiving these agents as part of their empiric therapy regimen. There was no significant difference in all-cause mortality or overall failure at end of therapy between the groups but nephrotoxicity was more common with additional glycopeptides (relative risk

1.88; 95% CI, 1.10–3.22). The investigators concluded that the use of glycopeptides in the treatment of patients with febrile neutropenia could be safely deferred until the documentation of a resistant gram-positive infection.[52]

Vancomycin is not currently recommended as standard initial antibiotic therapy for fever and neutropenia unless a patient has a possible catheter-related infection, skin or soft tissue infection, hemodynamic instability, or MRSA pneumonia.[2] Although several patients could meet these criteria, clinicians need to consider that if empiric vancomycin is started upon culture results, and if evidence of gram-positive organisms that require vancomycin therapy after 48 to 72 hours, it should be discontinued.

C. difficile Infection

Indirect effects of antimicrobial use include alterations in the normal intestinal microbiota creating a niche for C difficile infection (CDI).[53,54] Several studies have shown that risk for CDI is higher in HSCT and SOT recipients compared with other hospitalized and surgical patients, particularly in the setting of graft-versus-host disease, given the potential for damage to the gut luminal mucosa and the need for additional immunosuppression.[55] The incidence of CDI seems highest in the initial 3 months after SOT, with a peak at 6 to 10 days post-transplant.[56] Risk factors for CDI after SOT also include induction with antithymocyte immunoglobulin as well as after intensification of immunosuppression to treat graft rejection.[55–57]

Immunocompromised adults and children have several unique risk factors that may contribute to the severity of CDI. Independent of antibiotic exposure, cancer chemotherapy has been shown a risk factor and several agents have been implicated, including carboplatin, cisplatin, cyclophosphamide, doxorubicin, methotrexate, and topotecan as well as others.[53,54] Populations with underlying chronic comorbid conditions, including those with chronic kidney disease or HIV, also seem to be at increased risk of developing CDI.[54] It is not known whether these patients are at increased risk because of their underlying immunosuppression, their inability to develop an adequate immune response, exposure to specific medications, frequent exposure to antimicrobials, frequent and prolonged exposure to the health care environment, or a combination of these factors.[58] The diagnosis and management of CDI is a rapidly evolving topic.[59,60] It is not clear if immunocompromised hosts warrant different or longer courses of therapy compared with nonimmunocompromised hosts or if one therapeutic agent is superior to others. The decision to treat CDI with a specific agent should be based on severity of disease, balancing the risks and benefits of each regimen.

Limiting unnecessary exposure to antimicrobials is important in the prevention of CDI in immunocompromised patients. Opportunities exist to reduce not only unnecessary empiric antimicrobials but also the excessive duration of antimicrobial treatment.[15]

IMPLEMENTATION OF ANTIMICROBIAL STEWARDSHIP STRATEGIES FOR IMMUNOCOMPROMISED HOSTS

Antimicrobial stewardship for immunocompromised populations is most successful when a multidisciplinary team approach is used. Although a dedicated physician and pharmacist with knowledge of the complexities of infections in immunocompromised patients are necessary, a successful stewardship team also requires close partnership with physician champions on the oncology and transplant services. These physician champions can encourage their colleagues to adhere to the ASP guidelines and recommendations but are also important in updating the ASP team about unique infectious diseases risks with novel chemotherapeutic regimens. As proposed by Charani and colleagues,[59] to influence the antimicrobial prescribing of individual health care professionals, interventions need to address prescribing etiquette and use clinical leadership within existing clinical groups to influence practice. Understanding prescribers' attitudes, perceptions, and behaviors is particularly important when providing recommendations in immunocompromised patients.

The importance of a consistent stewardship team is particularly important to developing trust. Yeo and colleagues[52] demonstrated that antimicrobial stewardship strategies can be safely and effectively implemented with improved patient outcomes in the setting of hematology-oncology hospitalized patients, with dedicated ASP clinicians. In Yeo's study, when the ASP faced manpower limitations and dedicated personnel were switched to a program led by rotating infectious diseases trainees, a significant reduction was observed in the number of stewardship recommendations, acceptance of those recommendations and increased antimicrobial prescriptions. This study highlights that particularly that dedicated personnel increases compliance and acceptance with antimicrobial stewardship recommendations.

Most of the existing literature on antimicrobial stewardship strategies focuses on immunocompetent hosts. There is a small but growing body of literature in cancer and bone marrow transplants[26,27] but no dedicated studies in SOT recipients. Target opportunities for antimicrobial stewardship in immunocompromised hosts are summarized in **Box 2**.

Formulary Review

A fundamental component of antimicrobial stewardship is formulary review. Choices should reflect local infectious epidemiology in the context of the population cared for at each institution and avoid duplication. It should take into account the therapeutic efficacy, side effects and costs of each agent.[61] In cases of immunocompromised hosts, formularies should be reviewed for antimicrobials commonly used for post-transplantation infection prophylaxis (eg, *Pneumocystis jiroveci* pneumonia toxoplasmosis, cytomegalovirus, herpes viruses, and fungal infections). In addition, there should be review of drugs used for prophylaxis and treatment of neutropenic fever.[15]

Box 2
Opportunities for antimicrobial stewardship in immunocompromised hosts

- Produce and distribute to health care providers updated antimicrobial susceptibility trends for common organisms
- Formulary review
- Preprescription authorization
- Postprescription review and feedback
  - Monitoring drug interactions
  - Renal dosing optimization
  - Streamlining and discontinuation of unnecessary antimicrobials
- Antifungal stewardship
- Antiviral stewardship
- Develop multidisciplinary protocols, algorithms, and guidelines for the diagnosis, management, and prophylaxis of common infections
- Discuss microbiology, antibiotic use, and infection-related outcome data in multidisciplinary committees

The ASP should review opportunities to standardize formularies, optimize costs, and provide guidance for the appropriate use of antimicrobials within their health care system.

Preprescription Authorization

One of the core strategies of antimicrobial stewardship is the requirement of prior authorizations for select antimicrobials. Findings from a single-center, observational study demonstrated the feasibility and economic benefits of prior antimicrobial approval by a dedicated ASP team among immune compromised patients.[62] Standiford and colleagues[62] reported that utilization costs per 1000 patient days decreased from $44,181 at baseline to $23,933 at 7 years, mainly because of decreased use of antifungal agents in the cancer center related to ASP interventions. There were also cost savings seen in the transplant unit from $985,471 before the program was implemented to $647,068. Within 2 years after discontinuing the ASP, however, costs per 1000 patient days significantly increased to $31,658. In addition to cost savings, prior approval programs in cancer centers have been shown to play a potential role in controlling outbreaks of MDROs,[63] although drawing cause-and-effect associations in these studies is challenging.

Perhaps even more important than in immune competent patients, patients should be followed prospectively to determine the appropriate duration of the restricted antimicrobial approved and to monitor and avoid adverse events in those patients for whom an antimicrobial request was denied.

Postprescription Review

Prospective observational studies[64–66] have demonstrated the benefits and viability of implementing postprescription review and feedback in hematology-oncology units with dedicated personnel and resources to perform antimicrobial stewardship activities. Yeo and colleagues[65] investigated the outcomes of postprescription review targeting HSCT patients and reported trends toward reduced prescription of some but not all audited antibiotics (primarily third- and fourth-generation cephalosporins), achieving an 87% compliance with ASP recommendations. Failure to reduce overall antibiotic consumption may have been attributable to the inclusion of neutropenic patients who received broad-spectrum therapy until resolution of fevers and neutrophil recovery. No patient-related adverse outcomes were demonstrated in either study. These studies suggest that prospective audit and feedback can be safely implemented in the complex setting of hematology-oncology patients with a well-structured antimicrobial stewardship team. Improving patient care may not result, however, in overall decrease antimicrobial use, and ASPs should carefully consider the outcomes to be measured when any intervention is implemented.

Clinical Pathways and Compliance with Guidelines

Clinical pathways involve the development of peer-reviewed guidelines for the prevention or treatment of commonly encountered infections, simplifying the decision of antimicrobial selection.[61] Findings from single-center observational studies[67,68] demonstrated that developing and implementing clinical pathways for management of febrile neutropenia review can improve outcomes in hematology-oncology units. Pakakasama and colleagues[67] reported statistically significant reductions in septic shock, ICU admissions, and death compared with the period before implementation of such guidelines. Zuckermann and colleagues[68] reported in-hospital all-cause mortality was statistically significantly reduced compared with the preimplementation period. These improvements were seen despite only moderate compliance with 6 items in the clinical pathway (full compliance, 21.6%; partial compliance, 67.9%).

The development of clinical guidelines and pathways is not sufficient unless supplemented with proper education. Prior to their implementation, it is critical to ensure that important stakeholders have a chance to review the guidelines and the opportunity to provide feedback. When resources are available, ASPs should prospectively monitor compliance and provide feedback to prescribers when health care providers deviate from evidence-based recommendations. Examples of national guidelines relevant to immunocompromised hosts that could be adapted to each hospital setting include guidelines for the empiric treatment for fever and neutropenia[2,69,70] and the prevention of opportunistic infections in immunocompromised hosts.[71] Standardized order sets, order forms,[72] pocket cards, and computerized decision support tools can facilitate the implementation of guidelines and pathways.[73,74]

Antimicrobial De-escalation and Discontinuation

Recently published European guidelines for empiric antibacterial therapy for febrile neutropenic patients[49] recommend categorizing patients according to their risk for infections as candidates for antimicrobial escalation from those who will benefit from de-escalation. Decisions should be guided by the severity of clinical presentation, culture results, underlying disease, local epidemiology, and history of colonization.[49] Antimicrobial therapy could be discontinued despite persistent neutropenia in selected patients, depending on individual risk factors, expected bone marrow recovery, clinical symptoms, physical and radiologic findings, and negative laboratory results, including appropriate time for negative cultures. Such patients merit careful monitoring and a low threshold for resuming antimicrobial therapy.[75]

Based on limited observational studies, early discontinuation of antibiotic therapy while both fever and neutropenia persist was strongly discouraged for high-risk patients. In such cases, clinicians should search carefully for a potential infection source and change antibiotic coverage based on clinical or microbiologic evidence to add antifungal therapy empirically and/or should perform CT of the chest to search for invasive fungal disease.[2] As an alternative to prolonged hospitalization while waiting for bone marrow recovery, some centers switch patients who have defervesced to outpatient oral or intravenous regimens combined with careful daily follow-up.[76,77]

Appropriate dosing of antimicrobials based on the minimal inhibitory concentration of specific organisms[78] and adjustments according to variable volumes of distribution and hepatic or renal clearance are additional important activities for ASPs (see **Box 2**).

ANTIFUNGAL STEWARDSHIP

Antimicrobial stewardship has been traditionally focused on the judicious use of antibiotics and less attention has been given to antifungal agents. Antifungal agents are usually restricted in hospital formularies and often require the expertise of infectious diseases specialists or clinical pharmacists knowledgeable of the local epidemiology, susceptibility patterns, and current literature to guide appropriate prescribing.[30] Although emergence of resistant organisms is a less tangible problem than with antibiotics, it is of concern that there are only a few novel antifungal agents in development. Acquired antifungal resistance has been described for azoles in *Candida spp* and *Aspergillus spp*[79,80] and intrinsic resistance occurs in certain species eg, *Candida krusei* and fluconazole and *Scedosporium apiospermum* and amphotericin.[81] The high morbidity and mortality associated with invasive fungal diseases[82] and difficulties confirming a diagnosis contribute to the overuse of antifungal agents, including combination therapy and prolonged durations of therapies.[81,83]

Antifungal utilization can be optimized if health care providers use empiric, prophylactic, or preemptive strategies. Streamlining or de-escalation can be applied to all strategies applying evidence-based guidelines and ancillary diagnostic tests. In some institutions, the current practice is to start empiric antifungal therapy in patients with febrile neutropenia not improving on broad-spectrum antimicrobials[2] and in high-risk populations, such as patients with high-risk liver, intestinal[84] and lung[85] transplantation, acute myeloid leukemia, myelodysplastic syndrome, or allogeneic HSCT.[86,87] Other centers have used a diagnosis-driven approach within a clinical pathway prior to starting antifungal therapy.[88,89] The latter has proved safe in prospective cohort studies, allowing cost-effective and rational use of antifungals.[89] Screening high-risk patients with *Aspergillus* biomarkers or polymerase chain reaction (PCR) on a weekly or biweekly basis, in combination with reflex CT of the chest if the biomarkers or PCR are elevated, could avoid the unnecessary use of broad-spectrum antifungal agents, improving outcomes and decreasing hospital stay.[30,88,89] Appropriate dosing, monitoring drug interactions, and de-escalation of antifungals based on susceptibilities and appropriate control of the source of infection are also key functions of an ASP.[90,91]

ANTIVIRAL STEWARDSHIP

CMV is the most common viral infection after organ transplantation and has a significant impact on morbidity, mortality, and graft survival.[92] The diagnostic and therapeutic approaches to CMV prevention vary according to the transplanted organ and donor/recipient risks. Antiviral strategies and optimized dosing could be part of antimicrobial stewardship efforts to improve outcomes and minimize toxicities. International consensus guidelines on the prevention and treatment of CMV disease in transplant recipients recommend ganciclovir and valganciclovir as first-line therapy for prophylaxis and treatment of CMV infection and disease.[93] CMV immune globulins (CMVIG) is a product that was approved for prophylactic therapy of CMV disease in the 1980s. Historically, it was used for CMV prophylaxis based on 2 large clinical trials demonstrating benefit in kidney and liver transplant recipients. Both of these studies were conducted, however, against placebo and before ganciclovir was widely available for prophylaxis.[94] There are no published studies comparing the efficacy of CMVIG with antiviral therapy. Furthermore, all consensus guidelines state that there are few data to support the use of CMVIG when appropriate antivirals are given.[93]

RSV is a common cause of respiratory infections in children and immunocompromised adults with a high morbidity and potential mortality in HSCT recipients. Aerosolized ribavirin is the only approved drug by the Food and Drug Administration for treatment of high-risk infants with RSV; however it is commonly used in the treatment of immunocompromised adults with severe RSV infections. Publications on retrospective evaluation of HSCT have shown that preemptive treatment of upper respiratory tract infections with 5 to 7 days of inhaled ribavirin decreased progression to lower respiratory infections (47%–25%; $P = .01$).[95] Aerosolized ribavirin is, however, costly and cumbersome; thus, stratification of host risk has been suggested. Likewise, oral ribavirin was reportedly effective in small retrospective studies from lung transplant patients with good tolerance and effective response,[96] but another recent report found no differences in outcomes and bronchiolitis obliterans in lung transplant patients treated with oral and inhaled ribavirin.[97] Park and colleagues,[98] in a case-control study, compared oral ribavirin with placebo in the treatment of patients with hematologic disease patients with RSV, parainfluenza virus, or human metapneumovirus.

The 30-day mortality rate in the ribavirin group was 24% (5/21) versus 19% (4/21) in the nonribavirin group ($P = .71$). In addition, there was no difference in the 30-day adjusted mortality between the 2 groups. The potential costs, toxicities, and adverse events associated with the use of inhaled and oral ribavirin suggest that developing guidelines for the appropriate use of these agents could be a target for ASPs.

Other strategies in the prevention of RSV include the use of palivizumab, a monoclonal antibody designed to provide passive immunity. Cost-effective analysis of palivizumab has reported controversial results. Current recommendations support the use of palivizumab in certain high-risk children less than 2 years of age with chronic lung disease, congenital heart disease, and congenital neuromuscular and airway abnormalities, but the high cost versus benefits is not as evident outside of these indications.[99,100] Palivizumab prophylaxis or treatment palivizumab in stem cell transplant patients is not currently recommended. The drug has been used to control outbreaks,[101] but the cost-effectiveness of this intervention compared with other conventional infection control measures merits further investigation.

Literature on the use of immune globulins and monoclonal antibodies for the treatment or prevention of viral infections in immunocompromised hosts is controversial. ASPs could take the lead in developing guidelines, protocols, and algorithms in partnership with transplant and oncology teams for the appropriate use of immune globulins and monoclonal antibodies, prospectively monitoring patient-related outcomes to avoid expensive nonevidenced based practices.

RAPID DIAGNOSTIC METHODS IN ANTIMICROBIAL STEWARDSHIP

Diagnostic uncertainty could lead to the use of broad-spectrum antibiotics and prolonged courses of appropriate and inappropriately used antivirals. Traditional culture methods, such as blood cultures, have a decreased sensitivity if suboptimal volumes of blood are collected, lowering the yield of identifying the infectious organism and appropriately targeted antimicrobial therapy.[102] Optimizing the rapid diagnosis of infections could lead to the appropriate management of specific organisms and limit the use of unnecessary antimicrobials supporting antimicrobial stewardship efforts.[102,103]

These tests vary in methodology, ease of use, sensitivity, and specificity according to the assay but, in general, allow earlier recognition of the infectious agent compared with traditional culture methods. Prompt organism identification could lead to more timely appropriate selection of discontinuation of antimicrobial agents. With the use of yeast traffic light peptide nucleic acid–fluorescence in situ hybridization, 5 different *Candida* species and predicted susceptibilities patterns can be identified within 1.5 hours after growth, allowing prompt antifungal de-escalation from an echinocandin to an azole if the organism is susceptible.[104] Matrix-assisted laser desorption/ionization time of flight (MALDI-TOF) allows earlier identification of bacterial and fungal infections, decreasing the time to effective and optimal antimicrobial therapy,[105] providing important support to antimicrobial stewardship teams.[106] Perez and colleagues[105] found a reduction in length of hospital stay (11.9 vs 9.3; $P = .01$) and total hospitalization cost ($45,709 vs $26,126; $P = .009$) before and after the implementation of MALDI-TOF in combination with a strong antimicrobial stewardship team performing daily prospective audit and feedback to prescribers. Likewise, prospective multicenter nonrandomized studies have found that integrative pathways combining *Aspergillus* biomarkers, PCR platforms, and target radiologic evaluation facilitate earlier diagnosis and are cost effective in the diagnosis and management of invasive fungal infections in patients with hematologic malignancies.[107,108]

Respiratory virus diagnostic testing has also evolved in the recent years and is widely used in the diagnosis and management of children and immunocompromised patients. Multiplex PCR assays have higher sensitivity and specificity compared with rapid antigen testing and traditional culture methods for the identification of viruses, such as influenza, RSV, rhinovirus, adenovirus, CMV, and other viruses.[109] In addition, these support better infection control practices, allowing targeted cohort and isolation strategies[110] along with prompt initiation of antiviral therapy when indicated.

Rapid diagnostic tests are only of value when prescribers understand how to appropriately interpret and apply them.[108] ASPs should partner with local microbiology laboratories to determine which are the most appropriate diagnostic strategies for their patients and how to timely transmit those rapid results to the prescribers at bedside.

SUMMARY

Antimicrobial stewardship efforts in immunocompromised hosts are challenging due to the complexity of clinical scenarios, difficulties with accurate diagnosis, and the high mortality related to invasive bacterial, fungal, and viral diseases. Studies have demonstrated, however, that established stewardship strategies, such as prior approval and postprescription review, can be effective in this patient population. An enthusiastic, dedicated, multidisciplinary team with expertise in managing patients with various degrees of immunosuppression, along with input from providers primarily caring for these patients, is essential for a successful stewardship program.

REFERENCES

1. Poon LM, Jin J, Chee YL, et al. Risk factors for adverse outcomes and multidrug-resistant gram-negative bacteraemia in haematology patients with febrile neutropenia in a singaporean university hospital. Singapore Med J 2012;53(11):720–5.
2. Freifeld AG, Bow EJ, Sepkowitz KA, et al. Clinical practice guideline for the use of antimicrobial agents in neutropenic patients with cancer: 2010 update by the infectious diseases society of america. Clin Infect Dis 2011;52(4):e56–93.
3. Fishman JA. Infection in solid-organ transplant recipients. N Engl J Med 2007; 357(25):2601–14.
4. Marr KA. Delayed opportunistic infections in hematopoietic stem cell transplantation patients: a surmountable challenge. Hematology 2012;265–70.
5. Fishman JA. Infections in immunocompromised hosts and organ transplant recipients: essentials. Liver Transpl 2011;17(Suppl 3):S34–7.
6. Masterton RG. Antibiotic heterogeneity. Int J Antimicrob Agents 2010;36(Suppl 3): S15–8.
7. Theodoropoulos N, Ison MG. Current issues in transplant infectious diseases. Curr Infect Dis Rep 2013;15(6):453–4.
8. Oliveira AL, de Souza M, Carvalho-Dias VM, et al. Epidemiology of bacteremia and factors associated with multi-drug-resistant gram-negative bacteremia in hematopoietic stem cell transplant recipients. Bone Marrow Transplant 2007; 39(12):775–81.
9. Sifri CD, Ison MG. Highly resistant bacteria and donor-derived infections: treading in uncharted territory. Transpl Infect Dis 2012;14(3):223–8.
10. Martin SJ, Micek ST, Wood GC. Antimicrobial resistance: consideration as an adverse drug event. Crit Care Med 2010;38(Suppl 6):S155–61.
11. McGowan JE Jr. Economic impact of antimicrobial resistance. Emerg Infect Dis 2001;7(2):286–92.

12. Maragakis LL, Perencevich EN, Cosgrove SE. Clinical and economic burden of antimicrobial resistance. Expert Rev Anti Infect Ther 2008;6(5):751–63.

13. World Health Organization. The evolving threat of antimicrobial resistance. Options for action. World Health Organization. Available at: http://www.who.int/patientsafety/implementation/amr/publication/en/index.html. Accessed October 28, 2012.

14. Aitken SL, Palmer HR, Topal JE, et al. Call for antimicrobial stewardship in solid organ transplantation. Am J Transplant 2013;13(9):2499.

15. Tverdek FP, Rolston KV, Chemaly RF. Antimicrobial stewardship in patients with cancer. Pharmacotherapy 2012;32(8):722–34.

16. Dellit TH, Owens RC, McGowan JE Jr, et al. Infectious diseases society of america and the society for healthcare epidemiology of america guidelines for developing an institutional program to enhance antimicrobial stewardship. Clin Infect Dis 2007;44(2):159–77.

17. Clancy CJ, Chen L, Shields RK, et al. Epidemiology and molecular characterization of bacteremia due to carbapenem-resistant klebsiella pneumoniae in transplant recipients. Am J Transplant 2013;13(10):2619–33.

18. Cervera C, Linares L, Bou G, et al. Multidrug-resistant bacterial infection in solid organ transplant recipients. Enferm Infecc Microbiol Clin 2012;30(Suppl 2):40–8.

19. Shi SH, Kong HS, Xu J, et al. Multidrug resistant gram-negative bacilli as predominant bacteremic pathogens in liver transplant recipients. Transpl Infect Dis 2009;11(5):405–12.

20. Bergamasco MD, Barroso Barbosa M, de Oliveira Garcia D, et al. Infection with klebsiella pneumoniae carbapenemase (kpc)-producing k. Pneumoniae in solid organ transplantation. Transpl Infect Dis 2012;14(2):198–205.

21. Kalpoe JS, Sonnenberg E, Factor SH, et al. Mortality associated with carbapenem-resistant klebsiella pneumoniae infections in liver transplant recipients. Liver Transpl 2012;18(4):468–74.

22. Hammami S, Boutiba-Ben Boubaker I, Ghozzi R, et al. Nosocomial outbreak of imipenem-resistant pseudomonas aeruginosa producing vim-2 metallo-beta-lactamase in a kidney transplantation unit. Diagn Pathol 2011;6:106.

23. Abbo A, Carmeli Y, Navon-Venezia S, et al. Impact of multi-drug-resistant acinetobacter baumannii on clinical outcomes. Eur J Clin Microbiol Infect Dis 2007;26(11):793–800.

24. Schwaber MJ, Carmeli Y. Mortality and delay in effective therapy associated with extended-spectrum beta-lactamase production in enterobacteriaceae bacteraemia: a systematic review and meta-analysis. J Antimicrob Chemother 2007;60(5):913–20.

25. Gudiol C, Calatayud L, Garcia-Vidal C, et al. Bacteraemia due to extended-spectrum beta-lactamase-producing escherichia coli (esbl-ec) in cancer patients: clinical features, risk factors, molecular epidemiology and outcome. J Antimicrob Chemother 2010;65(2):333–41.

26. Gyssens IC, Kern WV, Livermore DM, et al. The role of antibiotic stewardship in limiting antibacterial resistance among hematology patients. Haematologica 2013;98(12):1821–5.

27. Averbuch D, Cordonnier C, Livermore DM, et al. Targeted therapy against multi-resistant bacteria in leukemic and hematopoietic stem cell transplant recipients: guidelines of the 4th european conference on infections in leukemia (ecil-4, 2011). Haematologica 2013;98(12):1836–47.

28. Bow EJ. Fluoroquinolones, antimicrobial resistance and neutropenic cancer patients. Curr Opin Infect Dis 2011;24(6):545–53.

29. Pepin J, Saheb N, Coulombe MA, et al. Emergence of fluoroquinolones as the predominant risk factor for clostridium difficile-associated diarrhea: a cohort study during an epidemic in quebec. Clin Infect Dis 2005;41(9):1254-60.
30. Ananda-Rajah MR, Slavin MA, Thursky KT. The case for antifungal stewardship. Curr Opin Infect Dis 2012;25(1):107-15.
31. Graffunder EM, Venezia RA. Risk factors associated with nosocomial methicillin-resistant staphylococcus aureus (mrsa) infection including previous use of anti-microbials. J Antimicrob Chemother 2002;49(6):999-1005.
32. Campillo B, Dupeyron C, Richardet JP. Epidemiology of hospital-acquired infections in cirrhotic patients: effect of carriage of methicillin-resistant staphylococcus aureus and influence of previous antibiotic therapy and norfloxacin prophylaxis. Epidemiol Infect 2001;127(3):443-50.
33. Weber SG, Gold HS, Hooper DC, et al. Fluoroquinolones and the risk for methicillin-resistant staphylococcus aureus in hospitalized patients. Emerg Infect Dis 2003;9(11):1415-22.
34. Liu WL, Chang PC, Chen YY, et al. Fluoroquinolone use and resistance of gram-positive bacteria causing healthcare-associated infections. J Antimicrob Chemother 2012;67(6):1560-2.
35. Bodro M, Gudiol C, Garcia-Vidal C, et al. Epidemiology, antibiotic therapy and outcomes of bacteremia caused by drug-resistant eskape pathogens in cancer patients. Support Care Cancer 2014;22(3):603-10.
36. Prabhu RM, Piper KE, Litzow MR, et al. Emergence of quinolone resistance among viridans group streptococci isolated from the oropharynx of neutropenic peripheral blood stem cell transplant patients receiving quinolone antimicrobial prophylaxis. Eur J Clin Microbiol Infect Dis 2005;24(12):832-8.
37. Yoo JH, Huh DH, Choi JH, et al. Molecular epidemiological analysis of quinolone-resistant escherichia coli causing bacteremia in neutropenic patients with leukemia in korea. Clin Infect Dis 1997;25(6):1385-91.
38. Rangaraj G, Granwehr BP, Jiang Y, et al. Perils of quinolone exposure in cancer patients: breakthrough bacteremia with multidrug-resistant organisms. Cancer 2010;116(4):967-73.
39. Lautenbach E, Strom BL, Bilker WB, et al. Epidemiological investigation of fluoroquinolone resistance in infections due to extended-spectrum beta-lactamase-producing escherichia coli and klebsiella pneumoniae. Clin Infect Dis 2001;33(8):1288-94.
40. Paterson DL, Mulazimoglu L, Casellas JM, et al. Epidemiology of ciprofloxacin resistance and its relationship to extended-spectrum beta-lactamase production in klebsiella pneumoniae isolates causing bacteremia. Clin Infect Dis 2000;30(3):473-8.
41. Garnica M, Nouer SA, Pellegrino FL, et al. Ciprofloxacin prophylaxis in high risk neutropenic patients: effects on outcomes, antimicrobial therapy and resistance. BMC Infect Dis 2013;13(1):356.
42. Irfan S, Idrees F, Mehraj V, et al. Emergence of carbapenem resistant gram negative and vancomycin resistant gram positive organisms in bacteremic isolates of febrile neutropenic patients: a descriptive study. BMC Infect Dis 2008;8:80.
43. Golledge CL, Carson CF, O'Neill GL, et al. Ciprofloxacin and clostridium difficile-associated diarrhoea. J Antimicrob Chemother 1992;30(2):141-7.
44. Weiss K. Clostridium difficile and fluoroquinolones: is there a link? Int J Antimicrob Agents 2009;33(Suppl 1):S29-32.
45. Charbonneau P, Parienti JJ, Thibon P, et al. Fluoroquinolone use and methicillin-resistant staphylococcus aureus isolation rates in hospitalized patients: a quasi experimental study. Clin Infect Dis 2006;42(6):778-84.

46. Gafter-Gvili A, Fraser A, Paul M, et al. Antibiotic prophylaxis for bacterial infections in afebrile neutropenic patients following chemotherapy. Cochrane Database Syst Rev 2012;(1):CD004386.

47. Roohullah A, Moniwa A, Wood C, et al. Imipenem versus piperacillin/tazobactam for empiric treatment of neutropenic fever in adults. Intern Med J 2013;43(10):1151–4.

48. Paul M, Shani V, Muchtar E, et al. Systematic review and meta-analysis of the efficacy of appropriate empiric antibiotic therapy for sepsis. Antimicrob Agents Chemother 2010;54(11):4851–63.

49. Averbuch D, Orasch C, Cordonnier C, et al. European guidelines for empirical antibacterial therapy for febrile neutropenic patients in the era of growing resistance: summary of the 2011 4th european conference on infections in leukemia. Haematologica 2013;98(12):1826–35.

50. Kim WJ, Weinstein RA, Hayden MK. The changing molecular epidemiology and establishment of endemicity of vancomycin resistance in enterococci at one hospital over a 6-year period. J Infect Dis 1999;179(1):163–71.

51. DiazGranados CA, Jernigan JA. Impact of vancomycin resistance on mortality among patients with neutropenia and enterococcal bloodstream infection. J Infect Dis 2005;191(4):588–95.

52. Paul M, Borok S, Fraser A, et al. Empirical antibiotics against gram-positive infections for febrile neutropenia: systematic review and meta-analysis of randomized controlled trials. J Antimicrob Chemother 2005;55(4):436–44.

53. Chopra T, Alangaden GJ, Chandrasekar P. Clostridium difficile infection in cancer patients and hematopoietic stem cell transplant recipients. Expert Rev Anti Infect Ther 2010;8(10):1113–9.

54. Dubberke ER, Burdette SD. Clostridium difficile infections in solid organ transplantation. Am J Transplant 2013;13(Suppl 4):42–9.

55. Tamma PD, Sandora TJ. Infection in children: current state and unanswered questions. J Pediatric Infect Dis Soc 2012;1(3):230–43.

56. Boutros M, Al-Shaibi M, Chan G, et al. Clostridium difficile colitis: increasing incidence, risk factors, and outcomes in solid organ transplant recipients. Transplantation 2012;93(10):1051–7.

57. Albright JB, Bonatti H, Mendez J, et al. Early and late onset clostridium difficile-associated colitis following liver transplantation. Transpl Int 2007;20(10):856–66.

58. Depestel DD, Aronoff DM. Epidemiology of clostridium difficile infection. J Pharm Pract 2013;26(5):464–75.

59. Charani E, Castro-Sanchez E, Sevdalis N, et al. Understanding the determinants of antimicrobial prescribing within hospitals: The role of prescribing etiquette. Clin Infect Dis 2013;57(2):188–96.

60. Brecher SM, Novak-Weekley SM, Nagy E. Laboratory diagnosis of clostridium difficile infections: there is light at the end of the colon. Clin Infect Dis 2013;57(8):1175–81.

61. Mihu CN, Paskovaty A, Seo SK. Antimicrobial stewardship: considerations for a cancer center. In: Safdar A, editor. Principles and practice of cancer infectious diseases. New York: Springer Science, Business Media; 2011. p. 491–8.

62. Standiford HC, Chan S, Tripoli M, et al. Antimicrobial stewardship at a large tertiary care academic medical center: cost analysis before, during, and after a 7-year program. Infect Control Hosp Epidemiol 2012;33(4):338–45.

63. Shaikh ZH, Osting CA, Hanna HA, et al. Effectiveness of a multifaceted infection control policy in reducing vancomycin usage and vancomycin-resistant enterococci at a tertiary care cancer centre. J Hosp Infect 2002;51(1):52–8.

64. Yeo CL, Wu JE, Chung GW, et al. Specialist trainees on rotation cannot replace dedicated consultant clinicians for antimicrobial stewardship of specialty disciplines. Antimicrob Resist Infect Control 2012;1(1):36.
65. Yeo CL, Chan DS, Earnest A, et al. Prospective audit and feedback on antibiotic prescription in an adult hematology-oncology unit in singapore. Eur J Clin Microbiol Infect Dis 2012;31(4):583–90.
66. Cosgrove SE, Seo SK, Bolon MK, et al. Evaluation of postprescription review and feedback as a method of promoting rational antimicrobial use: a multicenter intervention. Infect Control Hosp Epidemiol 2012;33(4):374–80.
67. Pakakasama S, Surayuthpreecha K, Pandee U, et al. Clinical practice guidelines for children with cancer presenting with fever to the emergency room. Pediatr Int 2011;53(6):902–5.
68. Zuckermann J, Moreira LB, Stoll P, et al. Compliance with a critical pathway for the management of febrile neutropenia and impact on clinical outcomes. Ann Hematol 2008;87(2):139–45.
69. Penack O, Buchheidt D, Christopeit M, et al. Management of sepsis in neutropenic patients: guidelines from the infectious diseases working party of the german society of hematology and oncology. Ann Oncol 2011;22(5):1019–29.
70. National Institute for Healthcare and Excellence. Neutropenic sepsis: prevention and management of neutropenic sepsis in cancer patients. Clinical guideline. Available at: http://publications.nice.org.uk/neutropenic-sepsis-prevention-and-management-of-neutropenic-sepsis-in-cancer-patients-cg151. Accessed November 14, 2013.
71. Guidelines for preventing infectious complications among hematopoietic cell transplant recipients: a global perspective. Bone Marrow Transplant 2009;44(8):453–558.
72. Cabrera-Cancio MR. Infections and the compromised immune status in the chronically critically ill patient: prevention strategies. Respir Care 2012;57(6):979–90 [discussion: 90–2].
73. Samore MH, Bateman K, Alder SC, et al. Clinical decision support and appropriateness of antimicrobial prescribing: a randomized trial. JAMA 2005;294(18):2305–14.
74. Madaras-Kelly KJ, Hannah EL, Bateman K, et al. Experience with a clinical decision support system in community pharmacies to recommend narrow-spectrum antimicrobials, nonantimicrobial prescriptions, and otc products to decrease broad-spectrum antimicrobial use. J Manag Care Pharm 2006;12(5):390–7.
75. DiNubile MJ. Stopping antibiotic therapy in neutropenic patients. Ann Intern Med 1988;108(2):289–92.
76. Horowitz HW, Holmgren D, Seiter K. Stepdown single agent antibiotic therapy for the management of the high risk neutropenic adult with hematologic malignancies. Leuk Lymphoma 1996;23(1–2):159–63.
77. Marra CA, Frighetto L, Quaia CB, et al. A new ciprofloxacin stepdown program in the treatment of high-risk febrile neutropenia: a clinical and economic analysis. Pharmacotherapy 2000;20(8):931–40.
78. Lortholary O, Lefort A, Tod M, et al. Pharmacodynamics and pharmacokinetics of antibacterial drugs in the management of febrile neutropenia. Lancet Infect Dis 2008;8(10):612–20.
79. Denning DW, Bowyer P. Voriconazole resistance in aspergillus fumigatus: should we be concerned? Clin Infect Dis 2013;57(4):521–3.

80. van der Linden JW, Snelders E, Kampinga GA, et al. Clinical implications of azole resistance in aspergillus fumigatus, the netherlands, 2007-2009. Emerg Infect Dis 2011;17(10):1846–54.

81. Cuenca-Estrella M, Alastruey-Izquierdo A, Alcazar-Fuoli L, et al. In vitro activities of 35 double combinations of antifungal agents against scedosporium apiospermum and scedosporium prolificans. Antimicrob Agents Chemother 2008;52(3): 1136–9.

82. Nivoix Y, Velten M, Letscher-Bru V, et al. Factors associated with overall and attributable mortality in invasive aspergillosis. Clin Infect Dis 2008;47(9):1176–84.

83. Yustes C, Guarro J. In vitro synergistic interaction between amphotericin b and micafungin against scedosporium spp. Antimicrob Agents Chemother 2005; 49(8):3498–500.

84. Brizendine KD, Vishin S, Baddley JW. Antifungal prophylaxis in solid organ transplant recipients. Expert Rev Anti Infect Ther 2011;9(5):571–81.

85. Avery RK. Antifungal prophylaxis in lung transplantation. Semin Respir Crit Care Med 2011;32(6):717–26.

86. Stanzani M, Battista G, Sassi C, et al. Computed tomographic pulmonary angiography for diagnosis of invasive mold diseases in patients with hematological malignancies. Clin Infect Dis 2012;54(5):610–6.

87. Cornely OA, Aversa F, Cook P, et al. Evaluating the role of prophylaxis in the management of invasive fungal infections in patients with hematologic malignancy. Eur J Haematol 2011;87(4):289–301.

88. Barnes RA, Stocking K, Bowden S, et al. Prevention and diagnosis of invasive fungal disease in high-risk patients within an integrative care pathway. J Infect 2013;67(3):206–14.

89. Barnes RA, White PL, Bygrave C, et al. Clinical impact of enhanced diagnosis of invasive fungal disease in high-risk haematology and stem cell transplant patients. J Clin Pathol 2009;62(1):64–9.

90. Shah DN, Yau R, Weston J, et al. Evaluation of antifungal therapy in patients with candidaemia based on susceptibility testing results: implications for antimicrobial stewardship programmes. J Antimicrob Chemother 2011;66(9):2146–51.

91. Apisarnthanarak A, Yatrasert A, Mundy LM. Impact of education and an antifungal stewardship program for candidiasis at a thai tertiary care center. Infect Control Hosp Epidemiol 2010;31(7):722–7.

92. Kotton CN. Cmv: prevention, diagnosis and therapy. Am J Transplant 2013; 13(Suppl 3):24–40 [quiz: 40].

93. Kotton CN, Kumar D, Caliendo AM, et al. Updated international consensus guidelines on the management of cytomegalovirus in solid-organ transplantation. Transplantation 2013;96(4):333–60.

94. Snydman DR, Werner BG, Heinze-Lacey B, et al. Use of cytomegalovirus immune globulin to prevent cytomegalovirus disease in renal-transplant recipients. N Engl J Med 1987;317(17):1049–54.

95. Shah DP, Ghantoji SS, Mulanovich VE, et al. Management of respiratory viral infections in hematopoietic cell transplant recipients. Am J Blood Res 2012;2(4): 203–18.

96. Pelaez A, Lyon GM, Force SD, et al. Efficacy of oral ribavirin in lung transplant patients with respiratory syncytial virus lower respiratory tract infection. J Heart Lung Transplant 2009;28(1):67–71.

97. Li L, Avery R, Budev M, et al. Oral versus inhaled ribavirin therapy for respiratory syncytial virus infection after lung transplantation. J Heart Lung Transplant 2012; 31(8):839–44.

98. Park SY, Baek S, Lee SO, et al. Efficacy of oral ribavirin in hematologic disease patients with paramyxovirus infection: analytic strategy using propensity scores. Antimicrob Agents Chemother 2013;57(2):983–9.

99. Joffe S, Ray GT, Escobar GJ, et al. Cost-effectiveness of respiratory syncytial virus prophylaxis among preterm infants. Pediatrics 1999;104(3 Pt 1):419–27.

100. Wang D, Bayliss S, Meads C. Palivizumab for immunoprophylaxis of respiratory syncytial virus (rsv) bronchiolitis in high-risk infants and young children: a systematic review and additional economic modelling of subgroup analyses. Health Technol Assess 2011;15(5):iii–iiv, 1–124.

101. Kassis C, Champlin RE, Hachem RY, et al. Detection and control of a nosocomial respiratory syncytial virus outbreak in a stem cell transplantation unit: the role of palivizumab. Biol Blood Marrow Transplant 2010;16(9):1265–71.

102. Afshari A, Schrenzel J, Ieven M, et al. Bench-to-bedside review: rapid molecular diagnostics for bloodstream infection - a new frontier? Crit Care 2012;16(3):222.

103. Laxminarayan R, Duse A, Wattal C, et al. Antibiotic resistance-the need for global solutions. Lancet Infect Dis 2013;13(12):1057–98.

104. Goff DA, Jankowski C, Tenover FC. Using rapid diagnostic tests to optimize antimicrobial selection in antimicrobial stewardship programs. Pharmacotherapy 2012;32(8):677–87.

105. Perez KK, Olsen RJ, Musick WL, et al. Integrating rapid pathogen identification and antimicrobial stewardship significantly decreases hospital costs. Arch Pathol Lab Med 2013;137(9):1247–54.

106. Tamma PD, Tan K, Nussenblatt VR, et al. Can matrix-assisted laser desorption ionization time-of-flight mass spectrometry (maldi-tof) enhance antimicrobial stewardship efforts in the acute care setting? Infect Control Hosp Epidemiol 2013;34(9):990–5.

107. Springer J, Morton CO, Perry M, et al. Multicenter comparison of serum and whole-blood specimens for detection of aspergillus DNA in high-risk hematological patients. J Clin Microbiol 2013;51(5):1445–50.

108. Holtzman C, Whitney D, Barlam T, et al. Assessment of impact of peptide nucleic acid fluorescence in situ hybridization for rapid identification of coagulase-negative staphylococci in the absence of antimicrobial stewardship intervention. J Clin Microbiol 2011;49(4):1581–2.

109. Kim H, Hur M, Moon HW, et al. Comparison of two multiplex pcr assays for the detection of respiratory viral infections. Clin Respir J 2013. [Epub ahead of print].

110. Mills JM, Harper J, Broomfield D, et al. Rapid testing for respiratory syncytial virus in a paediatric emergency department: benefits for infection control and bed management. J Hosp Infect 2011;77(3):248–51.

Hospital Antimicrobial Stewardship in the Nonuniversity Setting

Kavita K. Trivedi, MD[a],*, Kristi Kuper, PharmD, BCPS[b]

KEYWORDS

- Antimicrobial stewardship • Community hospitals • Small hospitals • Rural hospitals
- Long-term acute care hospitals

KEY POINTS

- Inappropriate antimicrobial use and antimicrobial resistance are problems that persist across the healthcare continuum.
- Several hospitals with limited infectious diseases resources have found ways to use available personnel to perform antimicrobial stewardship activities, with documented improvements in antimicrobial use and reductions in resistance and cost.
- Specific antimicrobial stewardship strategies are more feasible and effective in settings with limited infectious diseases resources.

INTRODUCTION

Regardless of the type of healthcare facility (large or small, urban or rural, academic or community) there is a 50% chance of a hospitalized patient receiving an antibiotic.[1] Studies have estimated that antimicrobial therapy is inappropriate and suboptimal 30% to 50% of the time for patients in acute healthcare settings.[2,3] Furthermore, inappropriate use of antimicrobial agents creates favorable conditions for resistant microorganisms to emerge, spread, and persist. To prevent the spread of antimicrobial resistance, US Centers for Disease Control and Prevention recommends every hospital optimize antimicrobial prescribing, also known as antimicrobial stewardship.[4,5]

Antimicrobial stewardship is a responsibility of all healthcare institutions, regardless of size,[6] to provide careful guidance and oversight of antimicrobials,[3] which can be provided through an antimicrobial stewardship program (ASP). An ASP promotes and measures the appropriate use of antimicrobial agents with the goals of minimizing adverse events, achieving optimal patient outcomes, limiting selective pressures that

Disclosure: Neither author has any relevant financial disclosures.
[a] Trivedi Consults, LLC, 1020 Curtis Street, Albany, CA 94706, USA; [b] VHA Performance Services, 521 East Morehead Street, Suite 300, Charlotte, NC 28202, USA
* Corresponding author.
E-mail address: kavita@trivediconsults.com

http://dx.doi.org/10.1016/j.idc.2014.01.007
0891-5520/14/$ – see front matter © 2014 Elsevier Inc. All rights reserved.

lead to the emergence of resistant organisms and *Clostridium difficile*, as well as reducing overall healthcare costs. An ideal ASP is a comprehensive system of multi-disciplinary healthcare providers, dedicated policies and procedures, and methods for data collection and outcomes reporting that promote optimal use of antimicrobial agents across the continuum of care. However, in many settings with limited infectious diseases expertise, information technology, and financial resources, these elements are not available because of lack of funding and/or personnel,[7] although programs have been developed and have prospered despite these barriers.

The ASP policy statement developed by the Society of Healthcare Epidemiology of America (SHEA), Infectious Diseases Society of America (IDSA), and Pediatric Infectious Diseases Society specifically recommends that the Centers for Medicare and Medicaid Services require all healthcare institutions (both inpatient and outpatient settings) to develop ASPs.[6] These ASPs are to be developed in accordance with the 2007 IDSA/SHEA guidelines and include a multidisciplinary team, antimicrobial formulary, institutional-specific guidelines for common infectious syndromes, interventions to improve antimicrobial use, facility-specific antibiograms, and processes to measure and monitor antimicrobial use.[3,6] Although developing a successful ASP is a challenge in any healthcare setting, there are unique challenges to hospitals with limited resources (eg, small, rural), where limited staffing and infrastructure may hamper the ability to implement ideal antimicrobial stewardship strategies. However, successful ASPs have been implemented in a variety of nonuniversity settings, and the experience with these efforts is instructive.

Most of the published data on antimicrobial stewardship in hospital settings comes from experiences in academic centers,[8-10] leading to a misconception that successful ASPs are only possible in settings with plentiful resources, including physicians and pharmacists with specialized training in infectious diseases (ID), personnel-in-training (eg, medical and pharmacy residents and fellows), informatics systems and technical support, and administrative support and funds. It is often assumed that healthcare settings with more limited resources (eg, community hospitals, small [fewer than 100 licensed beds] and/or rural hospitals), and long-term acute care hospitals (LTACHs) are incapable of supporting ASPs. However, it is useful to think of ASPs as a menu of interventions that are customizable and may be applied to any healthcare setting.[11]

A survey conducted in 568 US hospitals (most of which were community hospitals) indicates a diversity of resources available to implement ASPs.[11] Many of the components of an ASP may already be in place but not formalized. In a national survey of 406 hospitals antimicrobial stewards strategies such as guidelines/clinical pathways (66%) and parenteral-to-oral conversion protocols (64%) were reported in hospitals that did not consider themselves to have a formal ASP.[12] In a 2010 survey of pharmacy directors at 563 hospitals, 91% of respondents reported having a pharmacokinetic dosing program, and 84% had a mechanism in place to evaluate antibiotic use.[13] Staff pharmacists often perform these functions as part of their daily clinical activities, but other components of an ASP as recommended by the IDSA/SHEA guidelines may not be in place.[3] A 2011 national survey found that only 23% of community hospital ASPs were compliant with the IDSA/SHEA guidelines, compared with 55% of academic medical centers.[14] The most frequent barrier cited was lack of funding and/or personnel.

A mandate for processes encouraging the judicious use of antibiotics has existed for general acute care hospitals in California since 2008. In an assessment of 162 community hospitals in California conducted between 2010 to 2011, 49% reported an active ASP and 32% reported planning an ASP.[15] By beginning with efficient planning that focuses on problems or issues that can be addressed with available resources, effective ASPs are possible in the community hospital inpatient setting.

Community Hospitals

Community hospitals have been successful at implementing ASPs when they use targeted antimicrobial stewardship strategies and available personnel, and do not focus on the lack of ID expertise, if that is absent. One of the earliest published reports of an ASP in a community hospital documented the experience of a 120-bed hospital in Louisiana in 2003.[16] The ASP team consisted of an ID specialist, staff pharmacist, infection preventionists, and microbiologists. The team performed chart reviews 3 times per week. Total physician time invested in the ASP was between 8 and 12 hours per week. Patients receiving multiple, prolonged, or high-cost therapy were targeted. Notes or telephone calls were made to physicians if an intervention was recommended. The most frequent interventions were antimicrobial streamlining, conversions from parenteral to oral medications, and dose optimization. Over a 12-month intervention period, 488 recommendations were made, with an acceptance rate of 69%. Antibiotic costs declined from $18.21 per patient-day to $14.77 per patient-day (a reduction of 19%), which equated to total savings of $177,000. Although clinical outcomes were not formally evaluated, no adverse events were reported attributable to the ASP.

ASPs in community hospitals commonly begin on a smaller scale by evaluating antimicrobial usage patterns and resistance trends, and then devising interventions targeted at a single antimicrobial agent or class that is thought to be misused. For example, the use of fluoroquinolones as empiric therapy for *Pseudomonas aeruginosa* infections was the focus of a pharmacy-led ASP in a 565-bed, acute care, community teaching hospital in southern California.[17] This target is especially relevant because fluoroquinolones are the leading class of antimicrobial agents prescribed to adults in the US and fluoroquinolone resistance is a significant problem.[18] Components of this hospital's ASP included:

- Drug audits with post-prescription review and feedback
- Automatic intravenous (IV)-to-oral conversion programs
- A β-lactam–based institutional guideline for the treatment of *Pseudomonas aeruginosa* infections
- Educational programs targeting appropriate fluoroquinolone use

These interventions resulted in a 30% decrease in fluoroquinolone use since the inception of its ASP.[17]

Community teaching hospitals in Michigan and Toronto also used a drug-centric approach for their ASP initiatives. The Michigan program was composed of ID physicians and ID pharmacists who prospectively audited new antimicrobial starts and the weekly use of 8 target antimicrobials.[19] They showed significant reductions in *Clostridium difficile* rates, antimicrobial use, and pharmacy costs.[19] The program at the Canadian hospital was also composed of an ID physician and ID pharmacist and targeted a 12-bed intensive care unit, showing a reduction in antimicrobial costs and use of antipseudomonal agents with a prospective audit and feedback program in just 9 months.[20]

A perceived challenge for community hospital ASPs is the absence of both an ID physician and an ID pharmacist as per the IDSA/SHEA guidelines. In a national survey of smaller hospitals (80% with 25–300 beds), only 59% had an ID physician specialist on staff or available.[11] In another evaluation of 406 US hospitals, mostly nonteaching facilities, only 35% reported having an ID pharmacist.[12] Despite this resource limitation, there are reports of ASPs that have been implemented in community hospitals without dedicated ID resources. For example, a 236-bed acute care community hospital in Maryland established an ASP using existing clinical pharmacy resources with only remote access to an ID pharmacist for 16 hours per month.[21] An ID physician was consulted for administrative issues and shared chairperson responsibilities for the antimicrobial stewardship subcommittee, but no ID physician hours were dedicated to support daily ASP activities. The key components of the ASP included formulary restriction and prospective audit and feedback. Restricted antimicrobials were limited to prescription by an ID physician or intensivist (within the first 72 hours of admission) only. Patients receiving broad-spectrum antimicrobials were prospectively reviewed by a clinical pharmacist for appropriate use and streamlining potential. Automatic renal dose adjustment and IV-to-oral conversion was performed by staff pharmacists as part of the ASP. Data on select antimicrobials were gathered daily and aggregated quarterly for presentation to the antimicrobial stewardship subcommittee to identify trends. This information was also used in physician credentialing and communicated routinely to the Chief Medical Officer to improve physician compliance. Over a 2-year period, antimicrobial use, as measured by defined daily doses (DDD) decreased from 821.33 to 778.77 DDD/1000 patient-days ($P<.001$), resulting in $290,000 reduction in cost.[21]

Small Hospitals and Rural Hospitals

The composition of ASP teams that are responsible for day-to-day antimicrobial stewardship in small (fewer than 100 licensed beds) or rural hospitals is different from those of larger university-affiliated centers; consequently, the antimicrobial stewardship strategies that are feasible and effective in these hospitals may be different from those regularly implemented in other settings. ASPs in small and rural hospitals typically include staff pharmacists, infection preventionists and microbiologists, who often play multiple roles; infection preventionists may also function as laboratory directors, and pharmacists may also serve as clinical coordinators.[22] The pivotal role of staff pharmacists in ASPs in small or rural hospitals has been acknowledged.[23,24] When available, ID physicians are either members of the ASP team or serve as consultants, but more commonly hospitalists are involved because they are often the most frequent antimicrobial prescribers in community hospitals. Furthermore, hospitalists are ideally positioned to promote and lead antimicrobial stewardship efforts because they are leaders in many hospital-based quality-improvement initiatives.[25]

Limiting access to antimicrobials through formulary restriction is a primary strategy used in small and rural hospitals.[22] Formulary restriction limits the availability of multiple antimicrobial agents with overlapping spectra of activity, and also decreases drug purchasing costs. Other strategies commonly used in this setting include time-sensitive, automatic stop orders; dose optimization via automatic dose adjustments; and IV-to-oral antimicrobial conversion protocols. These are simple strategies that can be implemented by staff pharmacists on a regular basis.

Despite limited resources, small and rural hospitals can monitor outcome measures within their ASPs. In a Clostridium difficile infection (CDI) prevention/ASP project involving 8 small and rural hospitals in California, antimicrobial stewardship efforts were key in reducing healthcare–associated CDI rates.[22] Individual assessments were conducted for each hospital and so-called "low-hanging fruit" were identified for targeted implementation including identification of a pharmacy and physician champion, data mining of antimicrobial use to focus ASP criteria, and formulary restriction. Monthly conference calls were held over the course of a year to discuss best practices and provide expert consultation. At the conclusion of the study, healthcare–associated CDI rates decreased from 3.60/10,000 patient-days in the pre-intervention period to 3.23/10,000 patient-days in the post-intervention period (adjusted rate ratio, 0.68; 95% confidence interval, 0.17–2.67).[22] It was also recommended that the first 6 months to 1 year of each ASP serve as a pilot period, the results of which could be presented to administration for support and subsequently lead to the development of a formal ASP proposal.

Telemedicine provides healthcare over a distance via real-time audio and video conferencing to offer access to specialty care where it was previously unavailable, and it has also been used as a vehicle for enhancing antimicrobial stewardship activities. In a small, rural hospital in California, telemedicine services were used as a key component of the hospital's ASP.[26,27] The main tenets of the program included:

- Daily review of select antimicrobial orders by a pharmacist
- Daily phone calls between the pharmacist and the ID physician to identify cases requiring ID physician review
- Contact between the prescribing physician and ID physician to discuss flagged cases
- ID consultation via telemedicine (if requested by the prescribing physician or in the case of a difference in opinion)

Since 2008, this hospital's ASP has finalized the antimicrobial formulary, developed a system for pre-authorization for targeted antimicrobial agents, and implemented an IV-to-oral antimicrobial conversion program.[27] The ID physician and infection preventionist have conducted extensive educational programs, noon conferences, staff meetings, and case review conferences. The antimicrobial stewardship committee identified and focused on fluoroquinolone overuse, particularly for the treatment of cystitis and community-acquired pneumonia, resulting in a 77% reduction in fluoroquinolone use and an 80% reduction in overall fluoroquinolone pharmaceutical costs over a 4-year period[27] (Javeed Siddiqui, MD, MPH, personal communication, 2012).

Long-term Acute Care Hospitals

ASPs are also being implemented in LTACHs, which are specialty acute care hospitals that admit complex patients with acute care needs (eg, mechanical ventilator weaning, multiple comorbidities, need for IV antimicrobials, and complex wound care) and have a mean duration of stay of 25 days.[28] LTACH patients with multiple comorbidities have been shown to have high rates of healthcare–associated infections and multidrug-resistant organisms,[28] making the implementation of ASPs crucial. However, barriers may include a lack of clinical resources and/or commitment on the part of the LTACH to develop an ASP creating competing priorities in caring for extremely ill patients. A 2-person ASP team consisting of an ID physician and a clinical pharmacist in a 60-bed LTACH in Texas performed weekly post-prescriptive chart audits followed by feedback to prescribers.[29] After 15 months, clinicians had accepted 80% of ASP recommendations, resulting in a 21% reduction in antimicrobial use and a 28% reduction in cost per patient-day. An ASP team comprised of an on-duty hospitalist, an ID physician, a pharmacist, and an infection preventionist at an LTACH in northern California similarly conducted weekly rounds and reviewed all patients receiving 2 or more antimicrobials. Additionally, all patients receiving vancomycin or levofloxacin were also reviewed through the ASP because these antimicrobials were associated with the development of CDI in the LTACH (Debbie Wiechmann, RN, CIC, personal communication, 2011). The ASP team recommendations were communicated to the LTACH's quality review manager, who ensured that there was a follow-up review. Qualitative improvements in the use of antimicrobials in this medically complex patient population were documented.

Table 1
Strategies for implementing an ASP in a community or long-term acute care inpatient setting

Strategy	Examples
Education: key team members complete an antimicrobial stewardship educational offering	Society of Infectious Diseases Pharmacist Antimicrobial Stewardship Certification Program Stanford University Continuing Medical Education on https://www.coursera.org/course/antimicrobial Institution-specific pocket guides or empiric therapy guidelines disseminated to prescribers
Incorporate high-antimicrobial-prescribing physician disciplines into the ASP	Hospitalists Intensivists Emergency room physicians
Use nonphysician healthcare professionals as program extenders to assist with identifying inappropriate antimicrobial use	Nurses Case managers Pharmacy technicians Pharmacy or medical students
Develop, calculate and track a basic set of metrics related to antimicrobial cost and utilization that accounts for changes in patient census	Antimicrobial cost per adjusted patient-day Days of therapy per 1000 patient-days
Compile data summaries by department and track key parameters on a central scorecard	Multidrug resistant organism trends *Clostridium difficile* trends Pharmacist-directed antimicrobial interventions and acceptance rates Diagnostic testing practices
Prepare an annual antibiogram compliant with Clinical Laboratory Standards Institute guidelines[30]	Avoid duplicate patient isolates Do not report organisms for which there are fewer than 30 isolates Exclude surveillance cultures For small hospitals, consider aggregating data with healthcare facilities that share patients or with regional hospitals[31]
Allow staff pharmacists to make automatic conversions using guidelines approved by the Pharmacy and Therapeutics committee or other equivalent medical staff committee	Parenteral-to-oral conversions Renal dosing conversions Aminoglycoside and vancomycin dosing
Maximize information technology capabilities	Develop daily target drug lists that include pertinent laboratory information Include prompts in computerized physician order entry system to promote appropriate antimicrobial selection and identify indication for use Develop rules to identify organism-antimicrobial mismatches and repetition in spectra of activity (double coverage of anaerobes, gram-negatives, etc.) and patients with positive cultures not currently receiving antimicrobials Make antimicrobial duration of therapy visible at the point of care Evaluate the utility of clinical decision support systems

(continued on next page)

Table 1 (continued)	
Strategy	**Examples**
Evaluate diagnostic practices	Testing policy for urinalysis Rapid diagnostic testing and reporting processes Blood culture contamination rates Repeat testing of *Clostridium difficile* Antimicrobial susceptibility testing reporting practices, including selective reporting of susceptibility results to specific broad-spectrum agents
Incorporate evidence-based guidelines into order sets and protocols	Perioperative prophylaxis Community-acquired pneumonia treatment *Clostridium difficile* treatment Methicillin-resistant *Staphylococcus aureus* treatment

Where to Start

Developing an ASP in a setting with limited resources must begin with efficient planning and a thorough understanding of what is available. A good first step is to identify all interested parties, ideally starting with approaching the professionals outlined in the policy statement mentioned earlier. Hospital administration must be engaged from the outset. If support from hospital leadership is lacking, antimicrobial prescribers may be less likely to comply with recommendations from the ASP. Second, understand current institutional approaches for treating infectious disease syndromes, identify potential physician champions in the various subspecialties, evaluate available antimicrobial usage information, and review antimicrobial resistance trends. Then, devise interventions targeted at a single agent or class of antimicrobials that is being misused. Targeting 2 to 4 antimicrobial-related issues that can be addressed with available resources is more feasible than attempting to rectify all the institutional antimicrobial usage problems at once. Examples of other strategies to be considered are listed in **Table 1**. In addition, monitor at least one outcome and/or process measure per problem identified, at a minimum quarterly. Data collection helps to ensure the ASP is sustainable and will accumulate resources over time.

SUMMARY

Although it is well known that ASPs are effective in academic hospital settings with significant staffing and funding resources, successful antimicrobial stewardship is also possible in nonuniversity hospitals and may even be more critical in these settings. The development of ASPs in settings with limited resources where infectious diseases expertise, information technology, or financial resources may be lacking should be approached as a menu of interventions and strategies targeted to institutional needs and resource availability. Minimizing acquired resistance and improving patient outcomes decreases antimicrobial-related costs and supports the overall organizational goals that have to be achieved with limited means.

REFERENCES

1. Pestotnik SL, Classen DC, Evans RS. Implementing antibiotic practice guidelines through computer-assisted decision support: clinical and financial outcomes. Ann Intern Med 1996;124:884–90.

2. Cosgrove SE, Seo SK, Bolon MK, et al. Evaluation of postprescription review and feedback as a method of promoting rational antimicrobial use: a multicenter intervention. Infect Control Hosp Epidemiol 2012;33:374–80.
3. Dellit TH, Owens RC, McGowan JE Jr, et al. Infectious Diseases Society of America and the Society for Healthcare Epidemiology of America guidelines for developing an institutional program to enhance antimicrobial stewardship. Clin Infect Dis 2007;44:159–77.
4. Antibiotic Resistance Threats in the United States, 2013. Available at: http://www.cdc.gov/drugresistance/threat-report-2013/pdf/ar-threats-2013-508.pdf. Accessed November 4, 2013.
5. Fridkin SK, Srinivasan A. Implementing a Strategy for Monitoring Inpatient Antimicrobial Use Among Hospitals in the United States. Clin Infect Dis 2014;58(3):401–6.
6. Society for Healthcare Epidemiology of America, Infectious Diseases Society of America, Pediatric Infectious Diseases Society. Policy statement on antimicrobial stewardship by the Society for Healthcare Epidemiology of America (SHEA), the Infectious Diseases Society of America (IDSA), and the Pediatric Infectious Diseases Society (PIDS). Infect Control Hosp Epidemiol 2012;33:322–7.
7. Johannsson B, Beekmann SE, Srinivasan A, et al. Improving antimicrobial stewardship: the evolution of programmatic strategies and barriers. Infect Control Hosp Epidemiol 2011;32:367–74.
8. File TM Jr, Solomkin JS, Cosgrove SE. Strategies for improving antimicrobial use and the role of antimicrobial stewardship programs. Clin Infect Dis 2011;53:S15–22.
9. Lipworth AD, Hyle EP, Fishman NO, et al. Limiting the emergence of extended-spectrum beta-lactamase-producing Enterobacteriaceae: influence of patient population characteristics on the response to antimicrobial formulary interventions [abstract]. Infect Control Hosp Epidemiol 2006;27:279–86.
10. Fishman N. Antimicrobial stewardship. Am J Med 2006;119:S53–61 [discussion: S62–70].
11. Septimus EJ, Owens RC. Need and potential of antimicrobial stewardship in community hospitals. Clin Infect Dis 2011;53:S8–14.
12. Doron S, Nadkarni L, Price L, et al. A nationwide survey of antimicrobial stewardship practices. Clin Ther 2013;35:758–65.
13. Pedersen CA, Schneider PJ, Scheckelhoff DJ. ASHP national survey of pharmacy practice in hospital settings: prescribing and transcribing -2010. Am J Health Syst Pharm 2011;68:669–88.
14. Lusardi K, Kuper K, Coyle E, et al. Adherence to IDSA/SHEA antimicrobial stewardship guidelines: results of a nationwide survey [abstract 232]. Poster Presentation, IDSA Annual Meeting. Boston, October 21, 2011.
15. Trivedi KK, Rosenberg J. The state of antimicrobial stewardship programs in California. Infect Control Hosp Epidemiol 2013;34(4):379–84.
16. LaRocco A. Concurrent antibiotic review programs – a role for infectious diseases specialists at small community hospitals. Clin Infect Dis 2003;37:742–3.
17. Wong-Beringer A, Nguyen LH, Lee M, et al. An antimicrobial stewardship program with a focus on reducing fluoroquinolone overuse [abstract]. Pharmacotherapy 2009;29:736–43.
18. MacDougall C, Polk RE. Variability in rates of use of antibacterials among 130 US hospitals and risk-adjustment models for interhospital comparison. Infect Control Hosp Epidemiol 2008;29(3):203–11.
19. Malani AN, Richards PG, Kapila S, et al. Clinical and economic outcomes from a community hospital's antimicrobial stewardship program. Am J Infect Control 2013;41(2):145–8.

20. Leung V, Gill S, Suave J, et al. Growing a "positive culture" of antimicrobial stewardship in a community hospital. Can J Hosp Pharm 2011;64:314–20.
21. Michaels K, Mahdavi M, Krug A, et al. Implementation of an antimicrobial stewardship program in a community hospital: results of a three-year analysis. Hosp Pharm 2012;47(8):606–16.
22. Trivedi KK, Nennig M, Kazerouni NN, et al. Antimicrobial stewardship program development and enhancement in small hospitals and rural hospitals. California: 2011–2012. Poster Presentation, ID Week 2013. San Francisco, October 4, 2013. (abstract#1013).
23. American Society of Health-System Pharmacists. American Society of Health-System Pharmacists statement on the pharmacist's role in antimicrobial stewardship and infection prevention and control. Am J Health Syst Pharm 2010;67: 575–7.
24. Laible BR, Nazir J, Assimacopoulos AP, et al. Implementation of a pharmacist-led antimicrobial management team in a community teaching hospital: use of pharmacy residents and pharmacy students in a prospective audit and feedback approach. J Pharm Pract 2010;23:531–5.
25. Srinivasan A. Engaging hospitalists in antimicrobial stewardship: the CDC perspective [abstract]. J Hosp Med 2011;6:S31–3.
26. TeleMed2U. Available: http://www.telemed2u.com/html/about.html. Accessed March 30, 2012.
27. Siddiqui J, Kutz C, Large N, et al. A telemedicine based anti-microbial stewardship program. Oral Presentation, ID Week 2012. San Diego, October 18, 2012. (abstract#35273).
28. Munoz-Price LS. Long-term acute care hospitals [abstract]. Clin Infect Dis 2009; 49:438–43.
29. Pate PG, Storey DF, Baum DL. Implementation of an antimicrobial stewardship program at a 60-bed long-term acute care hospital. Infect Control Hosp Epidemiol 2012;33:405–8.
30. Analysis and presentation of cumulative antimicrobial susceptibility test data; approved guideline—third edition. CLSI document M39–A3. Wayne (PA): Clinical and Laboratory Standards Institute; 2009.
31. Tamma PD, Robinson GL, Gerber JS, et al. Pediatric antimicrobial susceptibility trends across the United States. Infect Control Hosp Epidemiol 2013;34:1244–51.

Transformation of Antimicrobial Stewardship Programs Through Technology and Informatics

Ravina Kullar, PharmD, MPH[a],*, Debra A. Goff, PharmD, FCCP[b]

KEYWORDS

- Antimicrobial stewardship • Technology • Informatics • Electronic health records
- Medical applications

KEY POINTS

- Antimicrobial stewardship programs (ASPs) are established to improve patient outcomes and simultaneously reduce overall costs and decrease antimicrobial resistance.
- Informatics and technology have made significant contributions in health care, which can enhance ASPs.
- Using electronic health records and clinical decision support systems to their potential as well as embracing medical applications (apps) and social media enable clinicians to improve antibiotic use.
- There is a need for a review of technology and informatics currently available to assist in ASPs.

INTRODUCTION

The Infectious Diseases Society of America (IDSA) and Society for Healthcare Epidemiology of America (SHEA) recommend that health care organizations invest in data systems capable of measuring quality improvement from antimicrobial stewardship implementation.[1] Successful antimicrobial stewardship programs (ASPs) have been shown to improve patient outcomes and decrease antimicrobial usage by up to 35%, with an annual savings to institutions of up to $900,000.[2–5]

Health care providers and the government are looking to informatics and technology to play an important role in managing costs, as well as improving health care

Conflicts of interest: Dr R. Kullar: employed by Cubist Pharmaceuticals and owns Cubist Pharmaceuticals stock. Dr D.A. Goff: serves on the Speaker's Bureau of Merck, Astellas, Nanosphere; received grants from Merck, Cubist, Astellas; serves on Advisory Board of Forrest, Cubist, Astellas, Rempex.

[a] Cubist Pharmaceuticals, Department of Medical Affairs, 55 Hayden Avenue, Lexington, MA 02421, USA; [b] Infectious Diseases, Department of Pharmacy, The Ohio State University Wexner Medical Center, 410 West 10th Avenue, Room 368, Doan Hall, Columbus, OH 43210, USA
* Corresponding author.
E-mail address: ravina.kullar@gmail.com

Infect Dis Clin N Am 28 (2014) 291–300
http://dx.doi.org/10.1016/j.idc.2014.01.009
0891-5520/14/$ – see front matter © 2014 Elsevier Inc. All rights reserved.

quality and patient outcomes. The Centers for Medicare and Medicaid Services (CMS) are embracing informatics by providing financial incentives to qualified institutions as they adopt, implement, upgrade, or show "meaningful use" of certified electronic health record (EHR) technology to improve patient care by meeting several predefined objectives established by the CMS.[6] By 2014, the federal government wants more than half of all health care institutions to use EHRs. Facilities that have not implemented EHRs by 2015 will be penalized. EHRs represent 1 role that technology plays in health care. Applications (apps) geared toward mobile computing devices (eg smartphones and tablets) have also made an increasing impact in health care.

The Secretary of Health and Human Services published a press release on May 22, 2013 entitled "Doctors and hospitals' use of health information technology more than doubles since 2012."[7] This press release highlights a survey by the Centers for Disease Control and Prevention (CDC), indicating that in 2008 only 17% of physicians were using an advanced EHR system versus more than 50% by the end of April, 2013.[8] Likewise, in 2008, 9% of hospitals adopted an EHR versus more than 80% receiving Medicare or Medicaid incentive payments for implementing, upgrading, or meaningfully using EHRs by the end of April 2013. The highest rates of meaningfully using EHRs have been among large (>400 beds) hospitals (77%), followed by small (100 beds) rural hospitals (76%) and medium (100–399 beds) (72%) hospitals. Although EHR adoption rates seem to have increased this past year, much of that came from practices that upgraded basic systems (which includes capabilities for ordering prescriptions, recording patient history and demographic information, recording a list of the patient's medications and allergies, recording patient problem lists, recording clinical notes, viewing laboratory results, and viewing imaging results) for meaningful use. The CDC data show that of the 72% of doctors using an EHR, about 40% were using a basic system that would not qualify for meaningful use incentives.[8] As these technologies become more widespread, they are increasingly being applied to efforts to improve antibiotic use. Therefore, the objective of this article is to describe the impact of informatics and technology, focusing on EHRs and clinical decision support systems (CDSSs), apps, electronic resources, and social media, on antimicrobial stewardship.

EHRS AND CDSSS
EHR Terminology

The Healthcare Information and Management Systems Society defines an EHR as "a longitudinal electronic record of patient health information generated by 1 or more encounters in any care delivery setting."[9] Various components are included in this information, such as patient demographics, progress notes, medications, vital signs, past medical history, immunizations, laboratory data, and radiology reports. An EHR has the capability to generate a complete record of a clinical patient encounter, as well as any other care-related activity directly or indirectly via interface, including evidence-based decision support, quality management, and outcomes reporting.

Several individuals in the health care system use the terms electronic medical record (EMR) and EHR interchangeably; however, these terms describe 2 different systems. EHRs rely on EMRs to be in place, and EMRs are less comprehensive than EHRs. Data in the EMR are a legal record of what happened to a patient during the course of their treatment at a care facility, allowing the health care practitioner to document, monitor, and manage a patient's treatment course at a facility.[9] In its simplest form, an EMR is a digital version of the traditional paper charts for an individual, which is limited to the health organization and cannot be shared. Unlike EMRs,

EHRs are created to extend beyond the health organization that originally collects the information. They contain information from all the clinicians involved in the patient's care and are built to share information with other health care individuals, including the patients themselves.

Three main associations create standards related to EHRs: Health Level Seven (HL7), Comité Européen de Normalisation–Technical Committee 215, and the American Society for Testing and Material E31. HL7 generates the most widely used health care–related electronic data exchange standards in North America and is used to send defined, encoded data from 1 application (such as the laboratory system) to another (such as the EHR).[9] The HL7 Electronic Health Records Special Interest Group was established in 2002 to "promote the uptake of EHR implementation by standardizing the functions that may be present, based on user selection, in an EHR-System."[10]

The Institute of Medicine has presented guidance on the main care delivery–related capabilities of an EHR system.[11] They identified 8 core functions that an EHR should have to improve patient safety, support delivery of effective care, facilitate management of chronic conditions, and improve efficiency. These core functions include health information and data, results management, order management, decision support, electronic communications and connectivity, patient support, administrative processes, and reporting and population health. HL7 then expanded these 8 core areas into a standard for certification required for participation in the CMS incentive programs, including panel management, clinical quality dashboards, and e-prescribing.[12]

EHR and CDSS Impact on ASPs

EHRs with an integrated CDSS, such as TheraDoc (Hospira, Lake Forest, IL) or SafetySurveillor (Premier, Charlotte, NC), have been shown to make the greatest contributions to enhancing ASPs. CDSSs are software that are able to identify patients requiring intervention via extracting data from various sections of the EHR, such as microbiology, drug, and laboratory data, to create alerts or reports in which the clinician can potentially intervene. CDSSs offer tools for automated, near real-time surveillance, alerting, and reporting, as well as integrating evidence-based medicine and clinical guidelines into the delivery of patient care.[13] CDSSs build on the foundation of an EHR and can be a stand-alone application or integrated into an EHR system. Several CDSSs are currently available geared toward aiding ASPs (**Table 1**).[14–20]

The first study to evaluate the impact of a CDSS on performance of a prospective audit with intervention and feedback was published by Hermsen and colleagues[21] at a 624-bed acute-care academic medical center. Before implementation of the CDSS (TheraDoc) in October 2008, there was no reliable way to identify patients for ASP intervention and no prospective audit with intervention and feedback. In the post-implementation period (September 2009–February 2010), patients were identified by generation of 8 types of alerts within TheraDoc. The antimicrobial stewardship-specific alerts included the use of multiple antimicrobials, redundant anaerobic coverage, drug-bug mismatch, use of vancomycin for coagulase-negative staphylococci or methicillin-susceptible *Staphylococcus aureus*, and receipt of antimicrobials in the absence of positive culture results. This study showed that implementation of the CDSS increased the number of intervention attempts, but a major disadvantage was the amount of time required by the ASP and information technology (IT) personnel to implement and maintain the system. Significant time was spent reviewing alerts (2–3 hours/day, with an additional 1–2 hours for interventions on actionable alerts and documentation). The investigators stressed the importance of ASP personnel working with vendors to reduce the number of nonactionable alerts.

Table 1
Third-party antimicrobial stewardship CDSS vendors

CDSS	Vendor	Key Features
SafetySurveillor	Premier, Charlotte, NC	Can be used to generate antibiograms: specific to user-designed time frames and units Integrated stewardship and infection control module Customizable work lists by user Includes access to training modules, cost justification letters, and so forth
TheraDoc Antibiotic Assistant	Hospira, Lake Forest, IL	Antibiotic Assistant: Tool for evidence-based recommendations Can be customized by individual user Integrated ability to track trends and document interventions Pager/e-mail alerts Creates antibiograms: unit, source, and time frame specific Data stored in on-site server
QC Pathfinder	Vecna, Cambridge, MA	Pharmacy and infection control component Pager/e-mail alerts Includes preprogrammed customizable alerts Customizable, real-time antibiograms Can store data on remote or on-site server
MedMined Surveillance Advisor	CareFusion, San Diego, CA	MedMined modules: Virtual surveillance infection: supports infection control activities Generates antibiograms Customizable alerts by user Evidence-based alerts preprogrammed E-mail alerts to users Clinical experts support team
Sentri7	Pharmacy OneSource, Bellevue, WA	Supports infection control and stewardship Relies on user-specific reports Creates institution-specific, annual antibiograms Started as tool for notating pharmacy interventions

Calloway and colleagues[22] measured the impact of the implementation of the CDSS TheraDoc into their 425-bed acute-care community hospital in Texas. Implementation of the new CDSS required decisions by pharmacists, clinicians, and the ASP. Although TheraDoc gives access to several alerts, the team chose to begin with 20 alerts, focusing on intravenous (IV) to oral conversion, renal dosing, and vancomycin use greater than 72 hours. The targeted alerts were directed at high-cost drugs and organisms that would cause harm to the patient if untreated or treated inappropriately. Overall, the department of pharmacy increased its clinical interventions from an average of 1986 per month to 4065 per month. The annual estimated cost savings after CDSS implementation was $2,999,508, representing a 96% increase per year and translating into a $1,469,907 annual return on investment.

Schulz and colleagues[23] developed an integrated CDSS tool, best practice alerts, using their third-party vendor software (SafetySurveillor) to make ASP recommendations in their EHR Epic (Verona, WI). The best practice alerts tool included the ASP recommendations, dedicated infectious disease (ID) clinical information derived from the EHR, antimicrobial orders, and optional educational links. A total of 1285 stewardship best practice alerts were created, and 249 (19.4%) were written for de-escalation in patients who remained hospitalized for at least 72 hours. Of the de-escalation recommendations, 69% were accepted and 12% were accepted with modifications within 72 hours. There was a significant decrease in total antibiotic consumption as well as in the use of broad-spectrum (anti–methicillin-resistant *Staphylococcus aureus* and antipseudomonal) agents, which occurred when recommendations were accepted compared with those rejected. The results from this study show that by creating a convenient, real-time CDSS tool integrated in the EHR, particularly Epic, there were improvements in appropriate antimicrobial usage. Several key features have been developed in Epic, including iVents (an Epic tool used to communicate and record ASP recommendations and interventions), antibiotic order forms and dose checking alerts, navigator (collates most of the ASP information needed to evaluate and make an educated decision regarding patient therapy into a single location, reducing the amount of user searching by centralizing the location of data and standardizing the variety of data presentation formatting) and best practice alerts, 96-hour stop date, patient scoring and monitoring, and IV to oral interchange to aid in the optimization of ASPs.[14]

Evans and colleagues[24] implemented a successful CDSS at Intermountain Medical Center in Salt Lake City, UT more than 20 years ago and reported significant reductions in excess drug dosages, antibiotic susceptibility mismatches, antimicrobial adverse events, and overall hospital costs. The University of Maryland Medical Center published the first randomized controlled study in 2006 evaluating the role of CDSSs in ASPs.[25] The investigators reported that with the support of a CDSS (PharmWatch, Cereplex, now SafetySurveillor, Premier), the ASP intervened on nearly twice as many patients as the control arm (359 vs 180 patients, respectively), and spent approximately 1 hour less each day performing stewardship activities. During the 3-month period evaluated, the medical center spent nearly $84,000 less on antimicrobials in the intervention group compared with the control group.

A CDSS tool, relying on diagnosis and treatment guidelines, designed as an EHR progress note, was implemented in 9 primary care practices to assist with the diagnosis of acute respiratory infections (ARIs).[26] The investigators created this tool to make recommendations to providers for further testing based on the patient's history and embedded treatment prompts regarding the appropriate use of narrow-spectrum antibiotics to treat ARIs. Broad-spectrum antibiotic usage for children and adults declined at an estimated 16%, a relative reduction of about 30% for adults and 45% for children during the 27-month intervention period.

EHR and CDSS Challenges

Although EHRs do have the potential to improve patient outcomes, a recent report[27] from the Research And Development Corporation surveyed 30 physician practices in 6 states, commissioned by the American Medical Association, to determine physicians' views on the current state of EHR technology. Characteristics of current EHRs that were most common areas of dissatisfaction included poor usability, time-consuming data entry, interference with face-to-face patient care, inefficient and less fulfilling work content, inability to exchange health information, and degradation of clinical documentation. However, physicians did approve of the concept of EHRs and valued having remote access to patient information and improvements in quality of care. Six in 10 physicians with EHRs stated that the technology improved the quality of care, with only 1 in 5 stating that they would prefer to use paper charts again. Overall recommendations by the investigators included improving physicians' knowledge base in EHRs, with better EHR usability being an industry-wide priority and a precondition for certification.

Moreover, in relation to ASPs, there are various limitations fundamental to EHRs and CDSSs. EHR and CDSS implementation requires a large financial commitment, skilled IT staff, leadership, and buy-in from physicians and administrators. Once implemented, coordinated care requires close integration of pharmacy and laboratory systems. Third-party CDSSs, when integrated into EHRs, can support the goals of ASPs; however, even with these systems, the ASP committee may still have to work with vendors to optimize the program. These CDSSs are expensive and range from $100,000 to $500,000 per year, depending on the size of the institution.[14] To use EHRs for ASP activities, hospitals should anticipate spending a significant amount of time customizing their system. In general, it may take up to 18 months of programming time for these resources to become available, including time to promote the need, create and validate the tools, and implement the system with ASP pharmacists and clinicians. Because of competing demands on IT department resources, a request might need to enter the hospital queue of CDSS requests, which prevents timely implementation of the ASP CDS system.[14] Compatibility problems with older systems may also delay implementation and optimization. Optimization of EHRs and CDSSs is often a trial-and-error process, requiring several adjustments to make the tools useful for ASPs.

ELECTRONIC RESOURCES AND SOCIAL MEDIA

In addition to CDSSs and EHRs, use of medical applications (apps) and eBooks has surged with the introduction of smartphones. With these technological advances, the steward can access a large amount of medical knowledge with the tap of a finger at the patient's bedside. However, connectivity alone does not affect patient care; how an app or an eBook is used is the true test.

Several medical schools across the United States are providing tablets to students, with many people complaining that they do not know how to effectively use this tool.[28] Part of this problem may stem from the fact that the senior educators never had this tool during their medical school training; therefore, the educator is learning at the same pace as the student. The developers of *Epocrates*, the number 1 downloaded medical app by physicians, surveyed physicians to inquire how they learned about new medical apps. The most common response from 60% of physicians was word of mouth from a friend.[29] The challenge of finding reliable accurate medical apps was highlighted in a recent publication.[30] The investigators reviewed more than 1200 ID apps from the Apple and Google Play stores to discover only 12 new apps that were developed by a health care provider, written in English, and easy to navigate.

Knowledge of the medical expertise involved in developing the app is crucial. Concerns about the accuracy of drug information within medical apps have resulted in significant changes in the approval process by Apple. Apple now requires that all drug dosing recommendations within an app have a reference. It is not clear if Apple has health care professionals cross-checking the accuracy of the references, but this change clearly portrays the potential negative impact on patient care if incorrect information is used to guide therapy. Despite these concerns, the value of having immediate access to information at the point of patient care has been game changing. In addition, this technology has provided tools for ASPs around the world.

Apps and Web Sites for Antimicrobial Stewardship

Several commonly used ID apps have been previously reviewed[30,31]; however, not all ID apps are applicable to antimicrobial stewardship. The *Johns Hopkins Antibiotic Guide, Sanford Guide, UpToDate,* and *Management of Candidemia* are examples of apps that can assist the steward in the day-to-day management of patients.

The *Johns Hopkins ABX Guide* (http://www.hopkinsguides.com) provides a thorough overview of most ID topics. Information can be searched by bug or drug. Uses that have not been approved by the US Food and Drug Administration (FDA) are included for each antibiotic, and practical clinical pearls are included for several diagnoses. This app is available on the iPhone, iPad, Android, and Blackberry devices.

The *Sanford Guide to Antimicrobial Therapy* (http://www.sanfordguide.com) also provides easy-to-search ID topics. Information can be searched by disease/condition, bug or drug information, therapeutic adjuncts, and tables. The activity table provides the spectrum of activity for all antibiotics. This table is especially useful for new or non–ID-trained stewards. This app is available for iPhone, iPad, and Android devices and has an annual fee of $29.99.

The comprehensive *UpToDate* (http://www.uptodate.com/home/product) clinical decision support resource released an app version for iPhone, iPad, Android, Windows Phone 8, and Windows 8 tablets. This point-of-care app provides evidence-based medical information, which is continuously updated. Many hospitals and health care systems provide on-site access to *UpToDate* online. The app version costs $499.00 annually.

Management of Candidemia in the Stewardship Era app provides evidence-based information on candidemia with respect to risk factors, diagnostic tests, collaborative management approaches, current etiologic trends, and the application of stewardship approaches. This app is free and is available for the iPhone and iPad (https://itunes.apple.com/us/app/management-candidemia-in-stewardship/id668650033?mt=8). Several institutions have developed ASP Web sites available to the public, some of which have been associated with significant cost savings.[32,33]

iBooks for Antimicrobial Stewardship

One of the authors of this article, Debra Goff, published a free iBook designed for the Apple iPad entitled *Infectious Diseases There's an App for That* (**Fig. 1**). The iBook is accessible in 51 countries and features 5 free ID-related apps (*Epocrates, IDPodcasts, Micromedex, Re-admit Risk,* and *Management of Candidemia*) to assist antimicrobial stewardship (https://itunes.apple.com/us/book/infectious-diseases/id686201907?mt=11). Unlike a written review article for a journal or an eBook, an iBook allows narrated video demonstrations to show the user how to navigate the app and apply it to stewardship activities. For example, most health care providers are not aware that within the resource center of the *Epocrates* apps (https://itunes.apple.com/us/app/epocrates/id281935788?mt=8), one has free access to the IDSA guidelines. The PDF of the guidelines may be downloaded to a smartphone or tablet for free. This is a valuable tool for ASP, particularly in resource-limited settings.

The *IDPodcast* app (https://itunes.apple.com/us/app/id-podcasts/id367837172?mt=8) is useful for stewardship physicians and pharmacists who need additional training in ID. More than 100 hours of *IDPodcasts* are provided by ID physicians and pharmacists on numerous ID topics. The steward may find the *Micromedex* app (https://itunes.apple.com/us/app/micromedex-drug-information/id390211464?mt=8) useful for quick antibiotic-specific dosing and monitoring. Unlike *Epocrates*, which lists only FDA-approved antibiotics indication and dosing, this app includes real-world dosing based on studies after FDA approval.

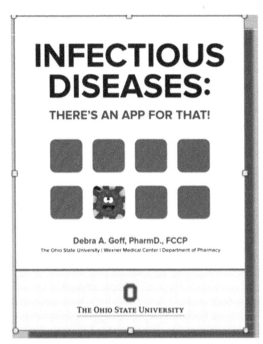

Fig. 1. Free iBook designed for the Apple iPad entitled *Infectious Diseases There's an App for That.* (*Courtesy of* Debra A. Goff, Columbus, OH.)

Twitter for Antimicrobial Stewardship

Since its inception in 2006, Twitter has become a social media tool for engaging with colleagues and monitoring ID developments in real time. Used wisely, Twitter can be a useful tool for stewardship physicians and pharmacists. Twitter can keep stewards up to date on ID news and literature locally and around the world. All major ID organizations such as the IDSA, National Foundation of Infectious Diseases, SHEA, and the CDC, use Twitter to stay connected to their members and to tweet ID topics of interest in real time. One can learn about outbreaks of flu or other ID topics first on Twitter since it is in real time. Many ID stewards Tweet links to articles or blogs. The ability to connect with other stewardship physicians and pharmacists worldwide on Twitter can be mutually beneficial. The user can follow organizations and specific people on Twitter without having to tweet, or the user can choose to become actively involved by sending tweets.

SUMMARY

With the increase of antimicrobial resistance and the dismal outlook for the antibiotic pipeline, effective ASPs in institutions are imperative. The government is now financially incentivizing institutions that have embraced technology, with the hopes of improving patient care and decreasing health care costs. EHRs and CDSSs have been shown to benefit clinicians in their daily ASP duties, as well as improve patient outcomes and decrease overall costs. However, for these technological advances to make the greatest impact, it is important for clinicians to be educated appropriately on EHRs and CDSSs. Likewise, although medical apps, iBooks, and Twitter may enhance stewardship activities, education is pivotal in maximizing the usefulness of these tools.

REFERENCES

1. Dellit TH, Owens RC, McGowan JE Jr, et al. Infectious Diseases Society of America and the Society for Healthcare Epidemiology of America guidelines for developing an institutional program to enhance antimicrobial stewardship. Clin Infect Dis 2007;44(2):159–77.
2. Carling P, Fung T, Killion A, et al. Favorable impact of a multidisciplinary antibiotic management program conducted during 7 years. Infect Control Hosp Epidemiol 2003;24(9):699–706.
3. Goff DA, Bauer KA, Reed EE, et al. Is the "low-hanging fruit" worth picking for antimicrobial stewardship programs? Clin Infect Dis 2012;55(4):587–92.
4. Ansari F, Gray K, Nathwani D, et al. Outcomes of an intervention to improve hospital antibiotic prescribing: interrupted time series with segmented regression analysis. J Antimicrob Chemother 2003;52(5):842–8.
5. MacDougall C, Polk RE. Antimicrobial stewardship programs in health care systems. Clin Microbiol Rev 2005;18(4):638–56.
6. Centers for Medicare and Medicaid Services. EHR incentive programs. 2013. Available at: http://www.cms.gov/Regulations-and-Guidance/Legislation/EHRIncentivePrograms. Accessed October 4, 2013.
7. Department of Health and Human Services. Doctors and hospitals' use of health IT more than doubles since 2012. Available at: http://www.hhs.gov/news/press/2013pres/05/20130522a.html. Accessed December 23, 2013.
8. Hsiao CJ, Hing E. Use and characteristics of electronic health record systems among office-based physician practices: United States, 2001–2012. Available at: http://www.healthit.gov/sites/default/files/onc-data-brief-7-december-2012.pdf. Accessed December 19, 2013.
9. National Institutions of Health. National Center for Research Resources: electronic health records overview. Available at: http://www.tree4health.org/distancelearning/sites/www.tree4health.org.distancelearning/files/readings/NCRR-EHROverview.pdf. Accessed December 19, 2013.
10. Dickinson G, Fischetti L, Heard S. HL7 EHR system function model: draft standard for trial use. Available at: http://www.providersedge.com/ehdocs/ehr_articles/HL7_EHR_System_Functional_Model-DSTU.pdf. Accessed December 19, 2013.
11. Institute of Medicine. Letter report 2003. Available at: http://www.nap.edu/catalog.php?record_id=10781. Accessed December 26, 2013.
12. Health Resources and Services Administration. Available at: http://www.hrsa.gov/healthit/toolbox/HealthITAdoptiontoolbox/QualityImprovement/whatarekeyfeaturesehr4qi.html. Accessed December 26, 2013.
13. Kaushal R, Shojania KG, Bates DW. Effects of computerized physician order entry and clinical decision support systems on medication safety: a systematic review. Arch Intern Med 2003;163(12):1409–16.
14. Kullar R, Goff DA, Schulz LT, et al. The "epic" challenge of optimizing antimicrobial stewardship: the role of electronic medical records and technology. Clin Infect Dis 2013;57(7):1005–13.
15. Birz S. Nurse Zone Web site. Available at: http://www.nursezone.com/nursing-news-events/devices-and-technology.aspx?ID=18768&Tab=1. Accessed December 23, 2013.
16. TheraDoc. TheraDoc Web site. Available at: http://www.stochasticaphelion.com/bungee/Build/products/abx_assist.html. Accessed December 23, 2013.
17. Hospira. Hospira Web site. Available at: http://www.hospira.com/products_and_services/clinical_software/theradoc/index. Accessed December 23, 2013.

18. Vecna. Vecna Web site. Available at: http://www.vecna.com/solutions/infection-surveillance. Accessed December 23, 2013.

19. CareFusion. CareFusion Web site. Available at: http://www.carefusion.com/medical-products/infection-prevention/surveillance-analytics/antimicrobial-stewardship.aspx. Accessed December 23, 2013.

20. Sentri7. Pharmacy One Web site. Available at: http://www.pharmacyonesource.com/images/sentri7/sentri7brochure.pdf. Accessed December 23, 2013.

21. Hermsen ED, VanSchooneveld TC, Sayles H, et al. Implementation of a clinical decision support system for antimicrobial stewardship. Infect Control Hosp Epidemiol 2012;33(4):412–5.

22. Calloway S, Akilo HA, Bierman K. Impact of a clinical decision support system on pharmacy clinical interventions, documentation efforts, and costs. Hosp Pharm 2013;48(9):1–9.

23. Schulz L, Osterby K, Fox B. The use of best practice alerts with the development of an antimicrobial stewardship navigator to promote antibiotic de-escalation in the electronic medical record. Infect Control Hosp Epidemiol 2013;34(12):1259–65.

24. Evans RS, Pestotnik SL, Classen DC, et al. A computer-assisted management program for antibiotics and other antiinfective agents. N Engl J Med 1998;338(4):232–8.

25. McGregor JC, Weekes E, Forrest GN, et al. Impact of a computerized clinical decision support system on reducing inappropriate antimicrobial use: a randomized controlled trial. J Am Med Inform Assoc 2006;13(4):378–84.

26. Litvin CB, Ornstein SM, Wessell AM, et al. Use of an electronic health record clinical decision support tool to improve antibiotic prescribing for acute respiratory infections: the ABX-TRIP study. J Gen Intern Med 2013;28(6):810–6.

27. Friedberg MW, Chen PG, Van Busum K, et al. Factors affecting physician professional satisfaction and their implications for patient care, health systems, and health policy; RAND Corporation. 2013. Available at: http://www.rand.org/content/dam/rand/pubs/research_reports/RR400/RR439/RAND_RR439.pdf. Accessed October 25, 2013.

28. Ma TP. Technology should not define medical education. Available at: http://www.kevinmd.com/blog/2013/10/technology-define-medical-education.html. Accessed September 1, 2013.

29. Wickland E. Epocrates study cites advantages to providers and patients in using drug reference apps. Available at: http://www.mhimss.org/news/epocrates-study-cites-advantages-providers-and-patientsusing-drug-reference-apps. Accessed September 1, 2013.

30. Moodley A, Mangino JE, Goff DA. Review of infectious diseases applications for iPhone/iPad and Android: from pocket to patient. Clin Infect Dis 2013;57(8):1145–54.

31. Burdette SD, Trotman R, Cmar J. Mobile infectious disease references: from the bedside to the beach. Clin Infect Dis 2012;55(1):114–25.

32. Gauthier TP, Lantz E, Heyliger A, et al. Internet-based institutional antimicrobial stewardship program resources in leading US academic medical centers. Clin Infect Dis 2014;58(3):445–6.

33. Sick AC, Lehmann CU, Tamma PD, et al. Sustained savings from a longitudinal cost analysis of an internet-based preapproval antimicrobial stewardship program. Infect Control Hosp Epidemiol 2013;34(6):573–80.

Antimicrobial Stewardship Interventions
Thinking Inside and Outside the Box

Keith W. Hamilton, MD*, Neil O. Fishman, MD

KEYWORDS

- Antimicrobial stewardship • Penicillin skin testing • Ward rounds
- Transitions in care • End of life • Multidisciplinary rounds

KEY POINTS

- Many health care facilities do not have antimicrobial stewardship programs in place.
- Antimicrobial stewardship ward rounds offer an efficient way to improve the acceptance of stewardship recommendations.
- Patients that report penicillin allergies often receive suboptimal treatment for infectious conditions so performing interventions to better identify those patients with true allergies, including penicillin skin testing, offer promise to providing more optimal care.
- Patient transitions in care from one health care setting to another result in errors and complications; therefore, improved antimicrobial stewardship in these transitions is essential.
- In addition to promoting centralized antimicrobial stewardship programs, leaders in stewardship should also promote judicious antimicrobial prescribing practices by all providers.

INTRODUCTION

Professional societies call for implementation of antimicrobial stewardship in all health care facilities, and provide detailed descriptions of optimal components and implementation strategies (**Table 1**).[1] However, less than 50% of acute and long-term care facilities in the United States perform regular stewardship activities.[2,3] The degrees to which these activities are performed are somewhat variable, and often proportional to hospital size and resources. It is not always clear how much impact these activities have on inappropriate antimicrobial prescribing practices. The most common barriers to implementation of stewardship interventions include lack of personnel, lack of financial resources, opposition from prescribers, and resistance from administration.[3] Because of the gap between guidelines and practice, health

Disclosures: Neither author has anything to disclose.
Healthcare Epidemiology, Infection Prevention and Control, Hospital of the University of Pennsylvania, Suite 101 Penn Tower, One Convention Avenue, Philadelphia, PA 19104, USA
* Corresponding author.
E-mail address: Keith.Hamilton@uphs.upenn.edu

Infect Dis Clin N Am 28 (2014) 301–313
http://dx.doi.org/10.1016/j.idc.2014.01.003   id.theclinics.com

Table 1	
Optimal components of a successful antimicrobial stewardship program	
Strategies	**Components**
Antimicrobial stewardship team	Hospital epidemiologist
	Clinical pharmacist with infectious diseases training
	Microbiologist
	Infection control practitioner
	Information technology specialist
Collaborative committees	Infection control committee
	Pharmacy and therapeutics committee
	Quality assurance
	Patient safety
Measurement capabilities	Information systems capable of measuring antimicrobial use
	Computer-based surveillance
Stewardship strategies	Preprescription authorization of select antimicrobial agents
	Prospective audit of antimicrobial prescriptions with feedback to prescribers
Supplemental strategies	Education
	Guideline development
	Specialized antimicrobial order forms
	Streamlining based on clinical and laboratory data
	Dose optimization
	Parenteral to oral conversion

care providers need to develop ways to leverage available resources and personnel to build and enhance antimicrobial stewardship programs, and to broaden the scope of antimicrobial stewardship.

To create a successful antimicrobial stewardship program, health care facilities, ambulatory practices, and patient care units need not fulfill all of the ideal components of a centralized stewardship program, but instead should focus on exploiting available assets most efficiently and effectively. Innovative strategies to accomplish these goals can take a variety of forms, ranging from advanced electronic alert systems to more simple interventions such as ward rounds with the antimicrobial stewardship team. These innovations can improve the efficiency and effectiveness of antimicrobial stewardship interventions, and can make antimicrobial stewardship a more universal and successful practice in all health care settings.

ANTIMICROBIAL STEWARDSHIP WARD ROUNDS

Many health care facilities have moved from a more tightly restricted system requiring preprescription authorization to a model that incorporates less restricted antimicrobial use up front but coupled with prospective audit and feedback, also know as postprescription review and feedback. Prospective audit and feedback to providers can be an effective method to improve judicious antimicrobial use. Many studies have shown significant reductions in inappropriate antimicrobial use, increases in cost savings, reductions in *Clostridium difficile* infection, and reductions in nosocomial infections with drug-resistant organisms.[4–7]

Many health care facilities performing prospective audit and feedback use phone calls or electronic messaging to deliver immediate feedback to prescribers.[8] Because factors that affect antimicrobial prescribing are complex, prospective audit is often not straightforward, and feedback to prescribers can be difficult and, therefore, unsuccessful. In these situations impersonal means of communication may be less effective. Some centers have used antimicrobial stewardship ward rounds as a method to more effectively change prescriber behavior. During these rounds, the stewardship team or individual members have face-to-face discussions with prescribers on the more challenging cases they review, as opposed to using less personal means of communication.

Ward rounds can serve many purposes simultaneously. When performed correctly, they can help increase the visibility of the stewardship team and facilitate the development of a more collegial environment. Antimicrobial stewardship teams may also build trust among patient care providers by providing real-time feedback and practical education, which medical education and adult learning studies have shown to be one of the most effective forms of education and behavioral change. These more personal means of communication are often more readily accepted than phone calls, which are often perceived as burdensome and interruptive. In doing so, they can serve to not only support postprescription review but also promote adherence with protocols and empiric treatment guidelines. The stewardship team can also more easily assist in making recommendations on correct dosing and diagnostic testing. Ward rounds can also allow stewardship personnel to more effectively recognize the barriers that prevent judicious antimicrobial prescribing. Finally, ward rounds are a more efficient and effective way of sorting through complicated cases, promoting compromise and consensus among stewardship personnel and individual prescribers.

Those health care facilities that have used antimicrobial stewardship ward rounds have demonstrated increased rates of acceptance of the stewardship team's recommendations when compared with less personal means of communication.[9] Some recommendations are more readily accepted than others. Recommendations that suggest dose changes, escalation of therapy, or changes to drugs within a similar spectrum are much more readily accepted than those that suggest de-escalation or discontinuation. Ward rounds increase the acceptance of all of these recommendations, even the traditionally more challenging ones. If the stewardship team has limited time, however, rounds should focus on those patients for whom de-escalation or discontinuation of therapy is suggested. Telephone or electronic communication is still fairly effective at making the other types of interventions. Different methods of stewardship rounds have been implemented at various health care centers.[9,10] Some hospitals have even embedded stewardship personnel in multidisciplinary rounds with the patient care team. There are no rounding structures that are clearly better than others, but they are likely most effective when they involve a stewardship physician.

IMPROVING THE EFFICIENCY OF PROSPECTIVE AUDIT AND FEEDBACK

Prospective audit and feedback can be daunting. The rate of inappropriate antibiotic use is estimated to range between 14% and 43% of all prescriptions.[11] It is estimated that the average hospital uses 839 antibiotic days of therapy per 1000 patient-days; there are almost enough antibiotics for every hospitalized patient to receive a full daily dose of an antibiotic each day.[12] The ability to effectively identify patients for prospective audit and feedback has prevented many centers from performing this method of stewardship. Faced with this intimidating volume of antimicrobial use, how can the stewardship team identify the areas of inappropriate use? Two strategies can help facilitate the audit of antibiotic prescriptions and have the potential to make prospective audit and feedback more widespread and effective: the Pareto Principle and electronic alerts.

The Pareto Principle, or Law of the Vital Few, is an economic tenet asserting that approximately 80% of the outcomes result from only 20% of the potential causes.[13] By focusing on these vital few, one can have an influence over much of the outcomes with less effort. This principle has been shown to apply to areas outside economics and business, including health care. In outbreaks, particular patients transmit the infection to disproportionately more secondary cases than other patients, the so-called super-spreader phenomenon.[14] The same dogma can be applied to antimicrobial stewardship, particularly to prospective audit and feedback. For health care facilities with limited resources, focusing efforts in areas where antimicrobial stewardship will achieve the most significant returns for the effort is essential.

With finite resources, health care facilities should focus efforts on the minority of conditions that represent most of the antimicrobial prescriptions and, ideally, that also represent most of the inappropriate antimicrobial prescriptions. Identifying the units, services, groups of providers, and even individual providers that represent significant proportions of inappropriate antimicrobial use is helpful when targeting audit and feedback. The process of identifying these target areas can vary based on available resources, but ideally should include discussion with infectious diseases consultants, chart audits of specific units or practices, and aggregate data collection and analysis of antimicrobial use and associated costs by service line, unit, or provider. However, the approach can be simplified based on available time and resources, and may simply involve collecting qualitative data from relevant medical personnel and focusing on common, often inappropriately treated infections such as community-acquired pneumonia, urinary tract infections, and skin and soft-tissue infections. Once the vital few are identified, prospective audit becomes more manageable, but will still have substantial effects on overall inappropriate antimicrobial use.

The second method to facilitate prospective audit and feedback is electronic alerts. The interested reader is referred to the article by Kullar and Goff in this issue for a more detailed account of the role of informatics in enhancing antimicrobial stewardship efforts. Medical informatics can also be used to create electronic alerts for stewardship personnel. Many centers that perform prospective audit and feedback rely on manual chart review to identify potential interventions. Before 2012 most hospitals used paper-based medical record systems, but the shift from paper to digital is moving quickly, and currently most hospitals in the United States use electronic medical record (EMR) systems.[15] This shift not only allows for more efficient review of patient medical records but also offers promise to allow the more efficient identification of inappropriate antibiotic used through electronic alerts.

Alerts to identify inappropriate antimicrobial use can be created within many EMR systems or within clinical surveillance software systems that many centers use for infection control surveillance and reporting. Providers interested in antimicrobial stewardship at health care facilities planning to shift to EMR systems, or with EMR systems currently in place, should advocate for the creation of these electronic alert systems. Electronic alerts can notify either patient care providers or stewardship personnel of potential interventions in real time (**Table 2**). At one institution, alerts directed at patient care providers have been successful at changing antimicrobial prescribing behavior.[16] Partnership with information technology staff at health care facilities is necessary to design these alerts within the existing EMR or clinical surveillance software system.

Some medical centers have begun to implement electronic alert systems, but this field is still in its infancy and only very preliminary research has been performed.[17–19] Nonetheless, as EMRs become more prevalent, the use of electronic alerts to facilitate antimicrobial stewardship offers promise to make prospective audit and feedback more efficient and comprehensive.

Table 2
Potential electronic alerts that can be implemented within EMR systems

Alert	Description
De-escalation	Identifies situations whereby antimicrobial therapy could be narrowed from broader-spectrum antibiotics to more narrow-spectrum antibiotics based on culture results
Bug-drug mismatch	Identifies situations whereby an organism is identified that is resistant to a patient's current antibiotic regimen
Unlikely infection	Identifies patients receiving antibiotics without any positive culture data or diagnostic testing within a defined period of time from initial antibiotic prescription
Inappropriate double coverage	Identifies inappropriate double coverage with repetitive antimicrobial spectra of activity
Parenteral to enteral transition	Identifies patients on intravenous agents that are highly bioavailable and could be administered orally
Drug dosing	Identifies drug prescriptions with doses that differ from recommended doses based on patient-specific factors such as weight and creatinine clearance

ANTIMICROBIAL STEWARDSHIP AND ANTIBIOTIC ALLERGIES

Often neglected but imperative considerations in antimicrobial stewardship are antibiotic allergies. Medication allergies are common, and of all antibiotic allergies penicillin is the most common, reported in 5% to 10% of patients.[20] When treated for infections, patients with reported penicillin allergies often receive broader-spectrum, suboptimal, and even more toxic agents than patients without reported penicillin allergies. In addition, many alternative agents to β-lactams such as vancomycin and aminoglycosides require intensive therapeutic drug monitoring, resulting in increased cost from laboratory testing and pharmacy monitoring. As such, reported penicillin allergy has been associated with increased antibiotic resistance, cost, length of hospital stay, and mortality.[21]

Only about 10% to 15% of patients with reported penicillin allergies actually have a positive reaction to penicillin skin testing.[21] Documenting a careful history can identify some nonallergic reactions to penicillin, as some patients report gastrointestinal intolerance or a family history of penicillin allergy as allergic reactions. Many of these inaccurate classifications can be perpetuated in the medical record if an accurate history is not obtained. Having stewardship or other hospital personnel document accurate histories on patients with reported penicillin allergy, and removing these allergies from the medical record when they do not represent true allergies, are essential to optimizing patient care.

Some reported allergies are more vague and difficult to classify despite careful history taking. Even if the previous reactions seem to resemble classic hypersensitivity reactions, most patients will still tolerate penicillin. In fact, true immunoglobulin E (IgE)-mediated reactions often wane over time, with only approximately 20% remaining allergic after 10 years.[21]

Penicillin skin testing can exclude IgE-mediated allergies and offers a novel way to increase optimal antibiotic use. Skin testing can be incorporated into stewardship team activities or in partnership with specialists in allergy and immunology. The skin-testing procedure should use major and minor determinants of penicillin, the by-products of penicillin that elicit allergic reactions.[21] Only major determinant reagents are available in the United States, so diluted penicillin G should be used as a substitute for the minor determinants. When used in conjunction, major and minor determinants have a negative predictive value of up to 99% for IgE-mediated allergic reactions. If skin testing is negative, a graded challenge with escalating doses of the antibiotic can be performed subsequently to further rule out penicillin allergy, particularly in patients who describe a more severe IgE-mediated allergic reaction. Penicillin skin testing should not be performed in patients with severe non–IgE-mediated reactions such as toxic epidermal necrolysis and Stevens-Johnson syndrome. The skin test cannot predict recurrence of these reactions, so an antibiotic suspected to have previously caused these reactions in any particular patient should be avoided. Consultation with a provider experienced in performing and interpreting penicillin skin testing should be undertaken before implementing this strategy of antimicrobial stewardship.

The use of penicillin skin testing has been shown to decrease the use of certain antibiotics, including vancomycin and fluoroquinolones, with no significant adverse reactions to patients, in addition to decreasing costs.[21] These findings have been replicated in various health care locations including ambulatory practices, inpatient units, intensive care units (ICUs), emergency departments, and preoperative settings.[21–26] Existing studies demonstrate the feasibility of implementation of penicillin skin testing in all of these settings using available personnel, including physicians, pharmacists, and other health care workers. Even health care facilities without extensive personnel resources can educate existing clinical staff to take relevant patient histories and perform penicillin skin testing when appropriate. Penicillin skin testing offers an innovative mechanism to enhance antimicrobial stewardship programs in all health care settings.

ANTIMICROBIAL STEWARDSHIP AT TRANSITIONS IN CARE

One area that has largely been excluded from stewardship interventions are transitions of care from one setting to another. It has long been recognized that patients are particularly vulnerable when they change from one patient care location to another or to home. Mistakes are often made when preparing a patient's discharge medications. These pervasive mistakes include incorrect dosage, incorrect therapeutic drug monitoring, incorrect duration, and incorrect medication choice. Furthermore, patients are often discharged on antibiotics even when the infection has been fully treated during the hospital stay.

With antibiotics specifically, duration is often inappropriate because many prescribers count the first day of discharge as the first day of antibiotics, although the patient may have been receiving a different but effective antimicrobial regimen while hospitalized. Discrepancies in antimicrobial prescriptions can also result in adverse events; up to 27% of all discrepancy-related adverse events occur after hospital discharge.[27] Therefore, simple medication reconciliation by unit-based pharmacists with reference to hospital treatment guidelines for choice, dose, and duration has the potential to have a significant impact on patient care by avoiding many of these discrepancy-related adverse events and decreasing the number of unnecessary days on antimicrobial therapy. There is little research in this area specific to antimicrobial agents.

Particularly susceptible to complications of antimicrobial therapy are those patients who are discharged on intravenous antibiotics either to home or to a subacute care facility. An increasing number of patients are being discharged on outpatient parenteral antimicrobial therapy (OPAT) as a result of the increasing prevalence of multidrug-resistant organisms. Unfortunately, there are significant complications associated with OPAT related to both the disease and the therapy itself. Complications of antibiotic use make up 19.3% of all visits to the emergency room for adverse drug events, and many antibiotics have to be discontinued because of adverse events, some of which are preventable with appropriate monitoring (**Table 3**).[28,29] Antibiotics are also frequent causes of renal injury, and the most common cause of drug-induced hepatotoxicity.[30] Catheters used to infuse intravenous antibiotics are also associated with nonnegligible risks of venous thromboembolism.[31]

Some antibiotics require frequent monitoring for therapeutic levels or toxicity to optimize treatment success and avoid adverse events. For instance, close pharmacy monitoring of drugs such as vancomycin and aminoglycosides are associated with more favorable outcomes. Those patients not monitored by pharmacy specialists have higher mortality (7% greater, $P<.0001$), longer lengths of stay (12% greater, $P<.0001$), higher expenditures (6% greater, $P<.0001$), more hearing loss (46% greater, $P<.0001$), and more renal impairment (34% greater, $P<.0001$) compared with those patients who receive appropriate monitoring.[32]

In addition, many severe conditions that were conventionally treated in the inpatient setting are being treated with OPAT (**Box 1**).[33] Many of these most common indications are associated with high rates of mortality, morbidity, and recurrence, even with the most careful clinical, laboratory, and radiographic monitoring. The rate and frequency of monitoring and degree of oversight of these patients varies significantly among different providers and health care facilities. When treatment and monitoring occurs in the home or in settings outside the health care facility primarily responsible for the patient's care, variations in care result, and the consequences of inappropriate treatment and monitoring become more apparent.

Unlike in the inpatient setting, oversight of patients on OPAT is decentralized, making intense oversight by individual medical providers challenging. Creation of a centralized service within a health care system to monitor patients on OPAT can result in significant improvements in process measures such as appropriate laboratory monitoring and follow-up. A dedicated physician or pharmacist trained in infectious diseases with physician oversight likely provides the best management.[34,35] Having a centralized monitoring service to ensure appropriate antibiotic selection, dosage, duration, and laboratory monitoring at and after discharge decreases the burden of individual medical providers seeing the patients for follow-up while standardizing monitoring and reducing variations in care.[35]

Table 3
Courses of selected antibiotics that are discontinued early owing to adverse events in patients receiving outpatient parenteral antimicrobial therapy

Antibiotic	Courses Discontinued Early (%)
Nafcillin	10
Oxacillin	8
Gentamicin	8
Clindamycin	8
Vancomycin	5
Cefazolin	4
Ceftazidime	4
Ceftriaxone	3

Data from Tice AD, Rehm SJ, Dalovisio JR, et al. Practice guidelines for outpatient parenteral antimicrobial therapy. Clin Infect Dis 2004;38:1660.

Box 1
Most common indications for outpatient parenteral antimicrobial therapy in order of frequency

Bone and joint infection (including spinal infection)

Endocarditis

Bacteremia (with or without central venous catheter)

Skin and soft-tissue infection

Prosthetic device infection

Intra-abdominal infection

Pneumonia

Central nervous system infection (meningitis, brain abscess, etc)

Surgical wound infection

Data from Chary A, Tice AD, Martinelli LP, et al. Experience of infectious disease consultations with outpatient parenteral antimicrobial therapy: results of an emerging infections network survey. Clin Infect Dis 2006;43:1292.

Some health care facilities have also required mandatory consultation from an infectious diseases specialist before discharge for patients with planned OPAT.[34,36] These centers have seen improvements in process measures, including optimization of antimicrobial regimens and improvements in outpatient follow-up with infectious diseases physicians. In fact, mandatory consultation before discharge resulted in a significant change in therapy in 52% of patients and discontinuation of intravenous antibiotics in 28% of cases, avoiding the potential adverse events associated with OPAT and potentially decreasing the risk of antimicrobial resistance.

Antimicrobial stewardship at the time of discharge or transitions in care offers promise to improve clinical outcomes, increase appropriate antimicrobial treatment, limit antimicrobial duration, decrease cost, and avoid preventable adverse events, thereby making a significant impact at a vulnerable time during patient care.

ANTIMICROBIAL STEWARDSHIP AT THE END OF LIFE

Hospice promotes palliative care for patients who are terminally or seriously ill, and provides a noble way for these patients to approach the end of life. This philosophy of medical care shifts focus from aggressive treatments and diagnostic procedures to comfort. In this setting, medications and procedures that do not align with this philosophy are discontinued. As in almost all other health care settings, however, antimicrobial agents are perceived differently from other medications and are often considered innocuous. This perception is multifactorial. Antimicrobial agents are one of the few medications that provide almost immediate cures for the medical conditions for which they are prescribed. Other common medical conditions such as heart disease, hypertension, and diabetes require indefinite courses of medical therapy, and the effects of not pursuing treatment are more nebulous. The effects of an untreated infection are often visually apparent and easily envisioned. Unlike chemotherapy and invasive medical procedures, antimicrobial agents often do not have direct adverse consequences of their use. Most patients who receive antimicrobial agents tolerate them without immediate incident.

Patients nearing the end of life are particularly susceptible to infections resulting from compromise of the normal physiologic barriers (skin breakdown, intravenous catheters, and urinary catheters), immunosuppression, and malnutrition. Both families and medical providers often equate infections to uncleanliness, so there is an entrenched aversion and compulsion to treat even when goals of care have shifted. In addition, some infections lead to patient discomfort, so their treatment can also be interpreted as palliative.[37] These competing factors and perceptions make the decision to use antibiotics at the end of life a complicated one. Therefore, it is not surprising that 27% of patients on hospice receive at least 1 antibiotic in the last 7 days of life.[38] Many hospice patients receive at least 2 antibiotics, and some receive up to 6 antibiotics in their last 7 days of life. The most commonly prescribed antibiotics are macrolides and fluoroquinolones, which comprise 75% of antibiotics.[39] Only 15% of patients receiving antibiotics in hospice care have a documented diagnosis of infection.[39]

The evidence of whether treating infections at the end of life actually improves symptoms is conflicting.[38–41] The strongest evidence for the use of antibiotics to improve symptoms in patients receiving palliative care is in those with symptomatic urinary tract infections. Patients treated for urinary tract infections report improvement in symptoms at a rate ranging from 60% to 92%, whereas patients with all other infectious diagnoses report benefit at more modest rates, if at all.[38] Although the adverse effects of antimicrobial use are often not immediate, there are many downstream consequences to both patients and society. Many patients acquire *Clostridium difficile* colitis, which can lead to additional morbidity and discomfort. From a societal and infection control perspective, patients treated with antibiotics at the end of life are more likely to acquire multidrug-resistant organisms (MDROs), and thus facilitate the spread of these organisms to other patients on the unit.[41] The lack of ability of providers to withdraw the use of antimicrobial agents at the end of life is independently associated with acquisition of MDROs.

It is appropriate to treat many patients with antibiotics at the end of life; therefore, antibiotic use should not be denied but should be consistent with the patient's and family's goals of care. The risks of antimicrobial therapy should be balanced against the marginal palliation they provide, especially for conditions other than symptomatic urinary tract infection. In addition, the same antibiotic restrictions and oversight provided to other patients should also be applied to this population.

STEWARDSHIP AT THE LEVEL OF PRESCRIBER OR UNIT

Guidelines and recommendations for antimicrobial stewardship have focused on the creation of centralized processes and infrastructure to promote judicious antimicrobial use (see **Table 1**). These programs generally require dedicated and trained personnel to regulate and monitor antimicrobial use. Many health care facilities lack resources and dedicated personnel to perform stewardship activities; therefore, stewardship is limited in most health care facilities. However, it may not be necessary to have significant dedicated resources to develop an effective stewardship program. To this effect, some interventions have focused on improving antimicrobial use at the point of patient care. Developing core generalizable practices for use at the point of care by front-line health care providers has the potential to facilitate judicious antibiotic use without additional personnel. The objective of such practices would be to help providers make appropriate decisions about when to start, stop, or change antimicrobials, and to encourage them to evaluate antimicrobial use on a daily basis.

Antimicrobial stewardship, at its core, is a quality improvement intervention and arguably the quintessential quality improvement initiative. Few quality improvement initiatives can claim decreases in hospital-acquired infections, antimicrobial resistance, and health care costs while simultaneously improving patient outcomes. Many other quality improvement interventions, such as infection control, have been transformed by decentralizing some of the responsibility, placing more emphasis on what individual providers and patient care units can do to prevent health care–associated infections through the use of checklists and bundles of best practices.

There are several practices fundamental to pragmatic antimicrobial prescription practices at the level of health care provider (**Table 4**).[42] Some hospitals have demonstrated that implementation of policies that require health care providers to use these best prescribing practices is feasible and sustainable, and positively affects adherence to clinical guidelines.[43] Doing so also facilitates prospective audit and feedback by stewardship personnel because of improved documentation. These best practices may be facilitated through the use of checklists or EMR systems. If provider-level best practices for antimicrobial prescribing are implemented, audit and feedback to prescribers on adherence to these practices are important to sustain the intervention. However, this process is facilitated by standardization of documentation, and can be performed in a more retrospective fashion.[43]

There are several examples of hospitalist-led stewardship efforts to improve antimicrobial prescribing at the point of care.[44] These efforts, including the implementation of evidence-based order sets, educational interventions, and periodic feedback, have been successful at improving clinical outcomes and decreasing cost. Future and ongoing collaboratives of hospitalists and stewardship within and among hospitals have considerable promise to improve antimicrobial prescribing behavior.

Certain units within the hospital may specifically lend themselves to such interventions. ICUs have high prevalence of antimicrobial use, with up to 71% of patients receiving antibiotics.[45] Moreover, these units often have the highest rates of antimicrobial resistance and *Clostridium difficile* infections, making stewardship interventions potentially more impactful. ICUs also have certain characteristics that may facilitate provider-level stewardship. Despite hospital size and resources, many ICUs have a multidisciplinary rounding structure and dedicated clinical pharmacists. These multidisciplinary rounds can facilitate the daily review of antimicrobial use and incorporation of best prescribing practices. There are also a discrete number of common conditions that, if targeted, represent at least 80% of antibiotic use in ICUs (urinary

Table 4
Fundamental antimicrobial prescribing practices

Time Period	Components
Initial prescription	Empiric treatment consistent with local and national treatment guidelines, and if not, sound reasoning is documented
	Appropriate microbiological and/or radiologic studies are obtained
	Indication for antimicrobial therapy is documented
Daily review of prescription	Review of results of microbiological and/or radiologic studies
	Streamlining of antimicrobial regimen based on result of studies when possible
	Discontinuation of antimicrobial agents when no longer necessary (appropriate duration, diagnosis of condition that does not require antimicrobial agents, etc)
	Parenteral to enteral conversion when appropriate

tract infection, pneumonia, sepsis, and surgical site/skin and soft-tissue infections), making guideline development and audit/feedback more facile.

Provider-level interventions have the potential to shift antimicrobial stewardship from a responsibility of administrators to a more universal practice among individual medical providers and patient care units, representing a culture change that other disciplines such as patient safety have seen transform their fields.

SUMMARY

Imprudent antimicrobial use is pervasive in the current health care environment. Relying on traditional methods of antimicrobial stewardship alone will not significantly limit inappropriate antibiotic use in the myriad health care settings. Identifying the areas where most inappropriate antibiotic use exists allows antimicrobial stewardship teams to leverage their resources most efficiently. Electronic alerts can broaden the scope of the audit process but also allow centers without significant resources to perform prospective audits more efficiently. To increase the effect of stewardship, the field also needs to include other nontraditional strategies, such as penicillin skin testing, to further promote judicious antibiotic use. Finally, to further curtail inappropriate antibiotic use, antimicrobial stewardship should be expanded to all areas of health care, and innovative strategies need to be developed so that antimicrobial stewardship becomes the responsibility of every health care provider.

REFERENCES

1. Dellit TH, Owens RC, McGowan JE Jr, et al. Infectious Diseases Society of America and the Society for Healthcare Epidemiology of America guidelines for developing an institutional program to enhance antimicrobial stewardship. Clin Infect Dis 2007;44:159–77.
2. Septimus EJ, Owens RC Jr. Need and potential of antimicrobial stewardship in community hospitals. Clin Infect Dis 2011;53:S8–14.
3. Pope SD, Dellit TH, Owens RC, et al. Results of survey on implementation of Infectious Diseases Society of America and Society for Healthcare Epidemiology of America guidelines for developing an institutional program to enhance antimicrobial stewardship. Infect Control Hosp Epidemiol 2009;30:97–8.
4. Doron S, Davidson LE. Antimicrobial stewardship. Mayo Clin Proc 2011;86: 1113–23.
5. Carling P, Fung T, Killion A, et al. Favorable impact of a multidisciplinary antibiotic management program conducted during 7 years. Infect Control Hosp Epidemiol 2003;24:699–706.
6. Fraser GL, Stogsdill P, Dickens JD Jr, et al. Antibiotic optimization: an evaluation of patient safety and economic outcomes. Arch Intern Med 1997;157:1689–94.
7. Solomon DH, Van Houten L, Glynn RJ, et al. Academic detailing to improve use of broad-spectrum antibiotics at an academic medical center. Arch Intern Med 2001;161:1897–902.
8. Tamma PD, Cosgrove SE. Antimicrobial stewardship. Infect Dis Clin North Am 2011;25:245–60.
9. Cairns KA, Jenney AW, Krishnaswamy S, et al. Early experience with antimicrobial stewardship ward rounds at a tertiary referral hospital. Med J Aust 2012; 196:34–5.
10. DiazGranados CA. Prospective audit for antimicrobial stewardship in intensive care: impact on resistance and clinical outcomes. Am J Infect Control 2012;40: 526–9.

11. Hecker MT, Aron DC, Patel NP, et al. Unnecessary use of antimicrobials in hospitalized patients: current patterns of misuse with an emphasis on the antianaerobic spectrum of activity. Arch Intern Med 2003;163:972–8.
12. Polk RE, Hohmann SF, Medvedev S, et al. Benchmarking risk-adjusted adult antibacterial drug use in 70 US academic medical center hospitals. Clin Infect Dis 2011;53:1100–10.
13. Juran JM. Quality-control handbook. New York: McGraw-Hill; 1951.
14. Braden CR, Dowell SF, Jernigan DB, et al. Progress in global surveillance and response capacity 10 years after severe acute respiratory syndrome. Emerg Infect Dis 2013;19:864–9.
15. Mathematica Policy Research, Harvard School of Public Health, Robert Wood Johnson Foundation. Health Information Technology in the United States: Better Information Systems for Better Care, 2013. In: DesRoches CM, Painter MW, Jha AK, editors. Princeton (NJ): Robert Wood Johnson Foundation; 2013. p. 9.
16. Schulz L, Osterby K, Fox B. The use of best practice alerts with the development of an antimicrobial stewardship navigator to promote antibiotic de-escalation in the electronic medical record. Infect Control Hosp Epidemiol 2013;34:1259–65.
17. Hermsen ED, VanSchooneveld TC, Sayles H, et al. Implementation of a clinical decision support system for antimicrobial stewardship. Infect Control Hosp Epidemiol 2012;33:412–5.
18. Huang Y, Reichley RM, Noirot LA, et al. Automated dose checking and intervention for bariatric patients. AMIA Annu Symp Proc 2007;983.
19. Resetar E, Reichley RM, Noirot LA, et al. Implementing daily dosing rules using a commercial rule base. AMIA Annu Symp Proc 2006;1073.
20. Charneski L, Deshpande G, Smith SW. Impact of an antimicrobial allergy label in the medical record on clinical outcomes in hospitalized patients. Pharmacotherapy 2011;8:742–7.
21. Unger NR, Gauthier TP, Cheung LW. Penicillin skin testing: potential implications for antimicrobial stewardship. Pharmacotherapy 2013;33:856–67.
22. Forrest DM, Schellenberg RR, Thien VV, et al. Introduction of a practice guideline for penicillin skin testing improves the appropriateness of antibiotic therapy. Clin Infect Dis 2001;12:1685–90.
23. Arroliga ME, Radojicic C, Gordon SM, et al. A prospective observational study of the effect of penicillin skin testing on antibiotic use in the intensive care unit. Infect Control Hosp Epidemiol 2003;5:347–50.
24. del Real GA, Rose ME, Ramirez-Atamoros MT, et al. Penicillin skin testing in patients with a history of beta-lactam allergy. Ann Allergy Asthma Immunol 2007;4:355–9.
25. Raja AS, Lindsell CJ, Bernstein JA, et al. The use of penicillin skin testing to assess the prevalence of penicillin allergy in an emergency department setting. Ann Emerg Med 2009;1:72–7.
26. Park M, Markus P, Matesic D, et al. Safety and effectiveness of a preoperative allergy clinic in decreasing vancomycin use in patients with a history of penicillin allergy. Ann Allergy Asthma Immunol 2006;5:681–7.
27. Boockvar K, Carlson LaCorte H, Giambanco V, et al. Medication reconciliation for reducing drug-discrepancy adverse events. Am J Geriatr Pharmacother 2006;4:236–43.
28. Shehab N, Patel PR, Srinivasan A, et al. Emergency department visits for antibiotic-associated adverse events. Clin Infect Dis 2008;47:735–43.
29. Chemaly RF, Barbara de Parres J, Rehm SJ, et al. Venous thrombosis associated with peripherally inserted central catheters: a retrospective analysis of the Cleveland Clinic experience. Clin Infect Dis 2002;34:1179–83.

30. Chalasani N, Fontana RJ, Bonkovsky HL, et al. Causes, clinical features, and outcomes from a prospective study of drug-induced liver injury in the United States. Gastroenterology 2008;135:1924–34.
31. Tice AD, Rehm SJ, Dalovisio JR, et al. Practice guidelines for outpatient parenteral antimicrobial therapy. Clin Infect Dis 2004;38:1651–72.
32. Bond CA, Raehl CL. Clinical and economic outcomes of pharmacist-managed aminoglycoside or vancomycin therapy. Am J Health Syst Pharm 2005;62: 1596–605.
33. Chary A, Tice AD, Martinelli LP, et al. Experience of infectious disease consultations with outpatient parenteral antimicrobial therapy: results of an emerging infections network survey. Clin Infect Dis 2006;43:1290–5.
34. Shrestha NK, Bhaskaran A, Scalera NM, et al. Contribution of infectious disease consultation toward the care of inpatients being considered for community-based parenteral anti-infective therapy. J Hosp Med 2012;7:365–9.
35. Keller SC, Ciuffetelli D, Bilker W, et al. The impact of an infectious diseases transition service on the care of outpatients on parenteral antimicrobial therapy. J Pharm Tech 2013;29:205–14.
36. Shrestha NK, Bhaskaran A, Scalera NM, et al. Antimicrobial stewardship at transition of care from hospital to community. Infect Control Hosp Epidemiol 2012;33: 401–4.
37. White P, Kuhlenschmidt H, Vancura B, et al. Antimicrobial use in patients with advanced cancer receiving hospice care. J Pain Symptom Manage 2003;25: 438–43.
38. Reinbolt R, Shenk A, White P, et al. Symptomatic treatment of infections in patients with advanced cancer receiving hospice care. J Pain Symptom Manage 2005;30:175–82.
39. Albrecht JS, McGregor JC, Fromme EK, et al. A nationwide analysis of antibiotic use in hospice care in the final week of life. J Pain Symptom Manage 2013;46: 483–90.
40. Vitetta L, Kenner D, Sali A. Bacterial infections in terminally ill hospice patients. J Pain Symptom Manage 2000;20:326–34.
41. Levin PD, Simor AE, Moses AE, et al. End-of-life treatment and bacterial antibiotic resistance. Chest 2010;138:588–94.
42. Cooke FJ, Holmes AH. The missing care bundle: antibiotic prescribing in hospitals. Int J Antimicrob Agents 2007;30:25–9.
43. Thakkar K, Gilchrist M, Dickinson E, et al. A quality improvement programme to increase compliance with an anti-infective prescribing policy. J Antimicrob Chemother 2011;66:1916–20.
44. Rohde JM, Jacobsen D, Rosenberg DJ. Role of the hospitalist in antimicrobial stewardship: a review of work completed and description of multisite collaborative. Clin Ther 2013;35:751–7.
45. Vincent JL, Rello J, Marshall J, et al. International study of the prevalence and outcomes of infection in intensive care units. JAMA 2009;302:2323–9.

Index

Note: Page numbers of article titles are in **boldface** type.

Infect Dis Clin N Am 28 (2014) 315–321
http://dx.doi.org/10.1016/S0891-5520(14)00023-3
0891-5520/14/$ – see front matter © 2014 Elsevier Inc. All rights reserved.

id.theclinics.com

Moving?

Make sure your subscription moves with you!

To notify us of your new address, find your **Clinics Account Number** (located on your mailing label above your name), and contact customer service at:

Email: journalscustomerservice-usa@elsevier.com

800-654-2452 (subscribers in the U.S. & Canada)
314-447-8871 (subscribers outside of the U.S. & Canada)

Fax number: 314-447-8029

Elsevier Health Sciences Division
Subscription Customer Service
3251 Riverport Lane
Maryland Heights, MO 63043

*To ensure uninterrupted delivery of your subscription, please notify us at least 4 weeks in advance of move.

Printed and bound by CPI Group (UK) Ltd, Croydon, CR0 4YY

03/10/2024

01040492-0013